# BRIDGING THE GAP
# FROM REHAB TO PERFORMANCE

# BRIDGING THE GAP
# FROM REHAB TO PERFORMANCE

## SUE FALSONE

### FOREWORD

### MARK VERSTEGEN

ON TARGET PUBLICATIONS
APTOS, CALIFORNIA

*Bridging the Gap from Rehab to Performance*

Sue Falsone

Foreword: Mark Verstegen

Illustrations by Danny Quirk unless otherwise noted, © 2018 Danny Quirk

Photographs by Christopher Barr unless otherwise noted, © 2018 Christopher Barr Photography

Athlete models: Kacie Flowers and Tristan Rice

ISBN-13: 978-1-931046-66-4
Second printing March 2019

On Target Publications
P O Box 1335
Aptos, California 95001 USA
*otpbooks.com*

Library of Congress Cataloging-in-Publication Data

Names: Falsone, Sue, 1974—author.
Title: Bridging the gap from rehab to performance / Sue Falsone; foreword
Mark Verstegen; preface Phil Sizer.
Description: Santa Cruz, California : On Target Publications, [2017] |
Includes bibliographical references and index.
Identifiers: LCCN 2017001348 | ISBN 9781931046664 (pbk. )
Subjects: LCSH: Sports medicine. | Sports injuries--Patients--Rehabilitation. | Performance.
Classification: LCC RC1210. F27 2017 | DDC 617. 1/027--dc23

LC record available at https://lccn. loc.gov/2017001348

# DISCLAIMER

This book is not a substitute for the medical advice of physicians. This information is meant to supplement, not replace, proper medical education or advanced-level training in strength and conditioning. Sports activity and athletic training poses inherent risks. The author and publisher advise readers to take full responsibility for the safety of their athletes. Before using the drills and interventions described in this book, make sure your equipment is well maintained. Do not impose risks beyond your athletes' level of experience, aptitude, training, and comfort level.

# DEDICATION

THIS BOOK IS DEDICATED TO MY MOM, LOUISE FALSONE,
FOR ALWAYS BEING THERE FOR ME THROUGH THIS CRAZY JOURNEY.

I COULDN'T HAVE DONE ANY OF IT WITHOUT YOUR LOVE AND SUPPORT.

# CONTENTS

# FOREWORD

It was 1999 and I was myopically focused on taking a vision of "Understanding and Upgrading Lives" through an individualized, proactive performance-based approach across the four pillars of sustainable high performance: Mindset, Nutrition, Movement and Recovery. We would focus on the top performers in the world, starting with professional athletes, then elite military and first responders, and finally population health.

The mission was simple, "To provide the finest performance systems, specialists, and platforms seamlessly integrated to efficiently and ethically enhance our athletes' performance." Athletes' Performance (now EXOS®) was born with no partners, no investors, and a relentlessly determined young me who was looking to build a multi-disciplined team of leading practitioners to move into our new award-winning facility in the heart of Arizona State University's athletic campus.

I was fortunate to have had deep relationships across the related areas of this field, including emerging global thought leaders in the PT/ATC worlds and sports medicine directors across professional and university sports. It would be critical to build the right multidisciplinary core team of highly collaborative, capable, and growth-minded professionals who were open to stepping into a new, seamlessly integrated model that would require their cross pollination across disciplines.

This open and growth mindset would be the most important attribute to making up our ONE Team in this young organization. This is why the recommendations of my respected peers were so important, and I focused on our ability to identify great people with high values and work ethics who were eager to add value in a pioneering and continuously improving organization.

Eventually, an exhaustive process of interviews with both established and young up-and-coming stars was nearly complete. The one outlier was a young PT/ATC who had just relocated from North Carolina to Arizona, who had been volunteering for us for a few months, and the team was really impressed by her. I didn't know much about her, but knew she deserved the opportunity as she was always positively interacting with all the various members of our team, and seemed to be contributing across all the areas of the EXOS.

On a Wednesday after the training and therapy sessions were completed, I got cleaned up and had a formal sit-down interview with Ms. Sue Falsone, PT/ATC. That moment, the next hour, and what has and will be a lifetime, we started a very focused, intense, and aligned discussion on all things "movement." Throughout our conversation, I learned of her amazing background working in team sports as a PT/ATC. I then wanted to know about the influential people and books in her life, her past difficult and positive experiences, her passions and dreams. My intensity in the conversation was equally matched by Sue's eagerness as I shared our EXOS vision and the mission necessary to help our clients achieve their goals.

Then came the discussion around movement and the need to "Bridge the Gap." This requires a seamless continuum of proactive care—not just reactive rehab, but getting upstream of the 70 percent of contributing factors to injury, decreasing pain, preventing pain, and helping every person perform at the highest level.

Finally, we got into the weeds about movement quality and the need for a holistic system of screening and cleaning dysfunctional movement patterns, even if it meant we had to "Isolate to Innervate to Integrate." We agreed on the importance of pillar strength as the foundation to "Position, Pattern, and Power." Sue was one truly impressive professional at 25, but what sane person would move all the way across the country without a prearranged job, so I had to ask. Her response was quick and precise "After researching you, the company, and the job description, I locked in the interview. WE have this. When do I start?"

That was the start, and this book, Bridging the Gap from Rehab to Performance is the ongoing journey to fulfill her responsibilities in serving her patients and performers and respected peers, all while moving forward with the greatest respect and humility.

Sue has worked very hard to earn a special perspective as a practitioner and a person—forged by the "EgoTestical" headwinds of sport, being the first female head athletic trainer in professional sport—from the early days of being the sole EXOS PT/ATC practitioner, seeing nearly every client daily.

She expected EVERYONE on our team to upgrade rather than jeopardize movement quality. The same was expected of Sue to truly understand from the table to the field, utilizing her movement and manual skills expertise. This truly defines Bridging the Gap, when each practitioner on a team has gone deep enough to understand and upgrade across the continuum of care, rather than being a bunch of people with degrees working in their divisions and handing people off with a smile.

I hope Bridging the Gap has greater meaning than just learning of the PT/ATC's role in the overall process. I hope it changes your expectations and perspective of what the future of health care holds. You should have the mindset that you—personally and professionally—are a powerful player in getting upstream to the majority of lifestyle-induced pre-disease and disease states.

By Bridging the Gap, you, Sue, and everyone you consider your peers will have made a difference for others to build on. Let's continue our shared journey to understand and upgrade lives through our collaborative culture as we accelerate quality outcomes for all.

Respectfully,
Mark Verstegen
President_Founder, EXOS®

# CHAPTER ONE
## FROM THE TABLE TO THE FIELD—
## WHY IS BRIDGING THE GAP SO IMPORTANT?

There are few things more daunting than helping a professional athlete go from injury through rehabilitation to performance. Here we have a person who has worked an entire life to reach the pinnacle of a sport, may be earning millions of dollars, and is carrying the championship hopes of a team and its fans.

Now it is up to us to help return these athletes to play. No pressure here!

Even if you do not work with professional athletes, to have people come to you in pain and unable to perform in their work or live their lives the way they want can be daunting. People in pain are often scared, do not understand the process of healing, and simply want to live life by their own standards. They come to you for answers.

Again, no pressure—it's just a person's quality of life being placed in your hands.

These are the scenarios that motivated me to write this book. My goal is to provide a practical guide for both clinicians and performance specialists to simplify the process necessary to get a client back to full health.

It does not matter whether your client is an All-Star pro, a weekend Joe, or anywhere between—the aim is for you to apply a patient-focused model that will not only get people back to full function, but more importantly, to full health.

We have a moral and ethical obligation to do nothing less, but in the process, a few things stand in our way.

Unfortunately, we are in a race to see how many letters we can put after our names, but our personal reputation and standing should be secondary at best. The main point of the degrees and qualifications should be furthering our education so we can apply knowledge to better serve our clients. That is not always the case. Sometimes, this letter chasing is more self-serving than patient focused.

We also have to stop thinking that our personal area of expertise is the be-all and end-all when it comes to client care—whether that be strength and conditioning, athletic training, physical therapy, or any other discipline. No matter how good you are and how effective your practice, you simply cannot go it alone.

Certainly, one person might be the quarterback for a certain stage of rehabilitation, such as a medical doctor after an athlete has had surgery.

Eventually the person in charge will hand the baton to another professional whose role is every bit as important in advancing the client's rehab.

This book will provide insight into how your specialty fits into the rehabilitation and performance continuum and hopefully will give you a deeper understanding of the significance of other complementary roles.

When we start delving into the different clinical and performance disciplines, we find that most professionals care about the same big-picture concepts, including assessment and evaluation, movement quality, and pain mitigation.

Once we cut through the terminology, it is clear that we have the same primary goal: to improve the wellbeing of the client. The best practitioners are those who try to be the best in their areas and at the same time recognize the important contribution of other specialties.

In preparing to teach a recent class on fascial techniques, I reread a book by Luigi Stecco, founder of the Fascial Manipulation® method, and noticed how, from the first page, he readily acknowledged the crossover of his work and the efforts of myofascial release and acupuncture experts. When we consider the "points," he is discussing, he acknowledges that many of them also overlap with Travell and Simons' trigger points; they overlap with acupuncture points, and some overlap with the motor points of a muscle.

Many people in Eastern and Western medicine, from the previous centuries through the present day, have an overwhelming similarity in areas of the body they consider important. The takeaway is that no discipline is better than another and that all have a place in the rehab spectrum.

When we are receptive to this interdisciplinary approach, we soon realize how well it fits into the human body of the clients we work with every day. Each system is wonderfully complex in its own right and each is interconnected with the others—from musculoskeletal, to nervous, to digestive, and beyond.

Just as we cannot isolate one part or system in the body, neither should we create disparate units that keep our professional disciplines apart, nor should we accept those that were previously established.

I hope that as you read this book, you are able to recognize where your strengths fit in a patient-centered bridging-the-gap model, and that you are humble enough to see those areas needing improvement in a new light. This can better inform the gaps in your care strategy and guide you in expanding your network to include professionals who are experts in the skills you do not currently have.

## FIRST, A WORD ABOUT THE BOOK ORGANIZATION

I envisioned the beginning of this book to speak more to the strength and conditioning specialist seeking more information about the rehabilitative aspect of the continuum. The latter chapters of this book are directed toward the clinical specialist who needs education on the performance phase of returning an athlete to sport.

Parts of the book will be more familiar to you than others depending on where you are in your career. There will also be a lot of overlapping information for all disciplines throughout the book.

The underlying goal is to bridge the gap between rehab and performance between the table and field…between professionals.

You might expect this book to flow smoothly from injury through tissue repair using orderly medical techniques in a linear fashion, such as:

*Assessing an injury*

*Initial therapies for tissue repair*

*Rehabilitation of an injury*

*Getting an athlete back on the field*

That is not how the rehab process works, as we will discuss along the way. Injury to recovery to return to play is not linear; it is a messy process and not at all predictable. Concepts overlap, professions overlap, and goals overlap. The steps we use often jump between categories as we move from the table to the field, so we will be covering the categories more broadly.

As you read certain chapters and sections, you might think, "That concept does not fit here. I think it should go in a different section of the book." I knew before even writing a word that this would be the case, and that your education, background, and experience will vary from mine and will create a different frame of reference. The "categories" are not absolute. The techniques that fall under each category are not absolute.

Where I have placed certain philosophies or techniques are simply my opinion and how I categorize things in my brain. If you categorize a technique, school of thought, or philosophy differently, that is totally fine. I want you to take away organizational concepts, not firm categorizations that may or may not fit into your belief system.

It is okay for us to disagree about where a concept or technique belongs in the continuum. There is overlap in every area this book touches on, and none of them fit exclusively in a particular bucket. Similarly, no single discipline owns a technique. I tried to offer my perspective of organization based on what I have done so far in my career and how I have seen things work well.

To provide opportunities for further reading and exploration, you will find a reference appendix to document the scientific research done on the topics covered in each chapter. It is important that we include an evidence-based element in our practices and use studies to inform our work.

However, that cannot be the only driving force. We need to remember that evidence-based practice (EBP) not only includes scientific evidence, but also clinician experience and takes into account patient values.

Clinician experience is classified as Level Five evidence, or mechanistic-based reasoning. It is made up of clinician observation and opinion. Although Level Five evidence is a low level of evidence, it is, nonetheless, a level of evidence. Our experiences and our scientific reasoning, based on science, are important as we navigate the world of EBP as it relates to clinical practice.

And our clinical experience, combined with the best available scientific evidence, means nothing if our plan doesn't align with the patient goals and values.

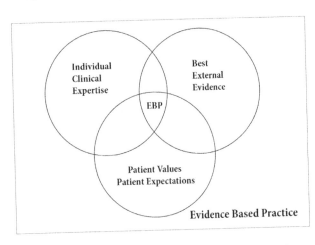

There is too much available information to find, prioritize, and put into action, which means it is all too easy to succumb to paralysis by analysis.

For example, if you went to a database like PubMed and searched for "neck pain," you would get tens of thousands of results. Even the most diligent person does not have time to sift through each one, read every study in its entirety, and come up with definitive conclusions about the various options for treating the cervical spine.

If you restricted your discovery to meta-analyses and systematic reviews,

you would still find that most of them tell us the studies conducted thus far are inconclusive and more research is needed before reaching a conclusion.

We need to admit that there is too much we do not know, whether we are talking about Western medicine principles like medications and exercise or Eastern techniques such as cupping and acupuncture. If we waited for everything to be validated by research, we would not get anything done, and our patients would not be treated.

## CLINICAL PEARL

Just because we don't know why something works, doesn't mean it doesn't work. We just haven't yet figured out the reason it works.

In my opinion, science, research, and evidence are three different things. I urge you to rely on evidence, but also realize we lack evidence in many areas of our practices. We have a lot of research on many subjects, but that research does not always point us in the same direction—if it did, we would have *evidence*.

In an absence of evidence or at least consistent research leading to similar conclusions, we can only turn to science to drive our clinical decision-making processes. Sometimes, interventions based on scientific theory are the best we can do.

There is nothing wrong with this. Research should be clinically driven, answer clinical questions, and drive us toward best practices. Clinical practice should drive research and then the evidence, after multiple research studies are performed in multiple populations takes us in the same direction and leads us to the best practice.

Our own experiences are also considered a level of evidence. It is a low level of evidence, but a level of evidence nonetheless. We need to take note of evidence-based best practices, but must also apply what we have seen manifest as practice-based evidence.

We should then freely share these insights, both within our specialties and to those in other disciplines so we can all take better care of our patients. That is the ultimate goal of *Bridging the Gap from Rehab to Performance*.

This is a complex process, and hopefully this book will provide some structure for you and your colleagues to collaborate in the best interest of the athlete, in the best interest of the patient…in the best interest of the client. Whatever words you choose to describe your working population, moving forward in this book, they will all mean the same thing.

Every person is an athlete in sport or life. Every athlete is a patient or client at some point. And every patient or client is a human being for whom we are trying to help improve quality of life.

## WHAT YOU WILL FIND IN THIS BOOK

We will touch on many different techniques and schools of thought. This is not a full resource outlining the intricacies

and details of each intervention. Instead, it will help you see where some of these fit within your current "bridging the gap from rehab to performance" model. It will also give you insight into how I organize my thought process when dealing with an injured athlete.

I have too much respect for everything in this book to do a discipline an injustice by claiming to fully represent the brand, school, or thought process. If something in this book piques your interest, pursue further education in that area.

This book would be volumes if we were to cover the amount of detail each of the strategies and interventions requires. You will find additional resources in Appendix Nine; I encourage you to seek more information from those sources.

As you go through the different sections of this book, think about the information being presented and decide what tools you have in your tool box that would fit in that section. You may see intervention options in one section, but may think that particular technique or school of thought should go into a different phase of the recovery. That is fine. The point of this material is to provide a framework to the thought process, not to be dogmatic about where therapies and techniques should go or how to organize them in your practice.

Once you decide what tools you will use to address the main factors of each section, you will begin to see where you focused your education and where your knowledge may need to have some holes filled. At the very least, this thinking will help you decide what professional relationships you need to cultivate for the betterment of your athletes.

For example, if you are a physical therapist (PT) who works with athletes in a clinic and do not have the opportunity to go into the weight room or be on the field, you should befriend an educated strength coach who can talk you through—and take your athletes through—the last sections of the book. Your athletes will need those skills to return to play.

And vice versa: If you are a strength coach who does not have the skills to put your hands on people, you should befriend a skilled manual therapist who can focus on the first two sections of the book—the pain generator and motion segments—to assist your athletes who are in pain.

This book is a guide to give structure to the artful practice of taking an athlete from the medical table to the field. As you know, no two athletes are the same. Everything and everyone is individualized. However, we need an organizational framework that repeatedly and successfully returns our athletes to play.

What we do is an art, and the art of what we do is what makes us unique clinicians who are able to interact with our clients. Our art is based on science, and science requires structure. It is my hope that this book can help any professional working in the sports rehabilitation and performance fields to bridge any gaps you may have in your personal practice.

## THE PERFORMANCE TRAINING CONTINUUM

Early on when I was with Athletes' Performance, now called EXOS®, we spent many days discussing the concepts of bridging the gap from rehab to performance. Defining this phrase, determining who was to be involved, and deciding how to best execute this with an injured athlete were our areas of focus, debate, and discussion.

We recognized that every professional had a place in the athlete-centered model; to assist the athlete to the best of our professional ability was and continues to be the goal. Although there may be different phases in this continuum, there is one common goal: to return the athlete to the field, possibly bigger, faster, and stronger than prior to the injury.

This concept permeates my entire thought process and career and allows me to collaborate with many remarkable professionals, learning from them and working together in the best interest of our athletes.

## REHAB, REHAB INTEGRATION, PERFORMANCE

When an athlete is injured, we need a quick and succinct diagnosis. Depending on the situation, the athletic trainer (AT) or the physical therapist (PT) may be the first person to see the injured athlete; however, often a referral to a medical doctor (MD) is warranted.

The MD's diagnosis is probably based on the athlete's account of what happened, objective testing including hands-on tests and any diagnostic assessments that might need to be performed, such as MRIs, CT scans, or X-rays.

Once the MD confirms a diagnosis, we create a game plan. This rehabilitation plan includes not only the MD and athlete, but also typically the AT or PT step in as well. The decision regarding surgery is made and rehab is planned accordingly.

During the rehab process, decreasing pain, managing swelling, regaining range of motion, and basic strength training for activities of daily living (ADLs) are the priority.

While the ultimate goal for an athlete is to return to the playing field, the immediate rehab focus includes restoration of ADLs and foundational movements such as gait and postural changes—such as sit to stand—if any are lacking.

Once these ADLs and foundational movements are restored or are at least being managed, an athlete can begin setting sights on loftier goals. Improving the overall strength, stamina, and body composition can be additional focuses, knowing that the ultimate goal is far greater than ADL performance.

We focus this time on restoring some of the general sport attributes that may have been lost during the rehab process. This area of rehab integration covers a lot of ground and leads directly into performance training.

Performance training focuses on all aspects of improving performance: moving at different angles, loads, and speeds that are necessary for a return-to-play scenario for an athlete. All aspects of performance training are necessary for proper return to play.

## EVALUATION, ISOLATE, INTEGRATE

A thorough *evaluation* provides an accurate diagnosis and establishes parameters in which to work during the rehab process. Without a full evaluation and the resultant diagnosis, we might miss critical information, which is often detrimental to the rehab progression.

Tissue-healing considerations are needed to ensure quality recovery from injury. We follow guidelines for tissue healing to repair tissue, giving the body the optimal environment to withstand the upcoming forces seen in rehab and performance training.

When we do not follow these tissue-healing guidelines, we often see re-injury during the return-to-play process or immediately upon return to the sport. An evaluation of and a respect for specific tissue-healing properties is vital in this process.

Once we have an evaluation, we begin the rehabilitation process, and here we are reminded that the concept of *isolation* is not about specific exercises. It is about body parts; when someone has a shoulder injury, we need to address the shoulder. That may seem implicit, but that is not always the case.

In this age of "functional training," we sometimes look too much at the big picture and not enough at the individual parts. A recovering shoulder must first have proper arthrokinematics, range of motion, and strength for ADLs if there is any hope of throwing a baseball. Tending to the injured body part and ensuring its function as a "part" is required before it can work as an element of the whole.

Finally, *integration* of that body part is needed in order to produce a high-level movement or even to perform most activities. We know the body does not operate in isolation and that one part will affect another. During this integrative phase, we emphasize the concept of kinetic linking for efficient performance of activities.

## DUTIES OF THE SPECIALISTS

In today's world, the roles of health care specialists are changing, with overlapping education, specialties, and duties based on education and workplace. No single profession owns any specific technique and skills often overlap between professions.

The following duty list should not pigeonhole a specialist into a certain area. Many modern specialists are working in non-conventional spaces, which will continue to improve our health care offerings to people across the board.

Where does rehabilitation end and performance training begin? Can this precise point be defined? Most of us in the rehab and training fields do not believe it can.

At all levels of our many roles—medical doctor, athletic trainer, physical therapist, strength and conditioning coach, and many more—returning an athlete to play after an injury is a continuum. There are no defined milestones for official hand-offs or timelines determining when an athlete has finished rehab and is beginning performance training.

Each person involved in the process of returning an athlete to full sports performance needs to understand the other professionals involved in the process, and should respect what each specialty brings to the table to help get that athlete back to play.

When professionals do not understand the educational background of other professionals, there can be an inherent distrust when passing off an athlete to someone thought to be less educated.

These misunderstandings lead to disdain, distrust, and disruption of communication. People fear that sharing athletes or asking for help is a sign of not knowing everything and is therefore a weakness that will result in lost business in the future. People try to work in silos, not wanting to collaborate for fear of being "found out" that they cannot do it all.

We cannot be everything for everyone in any aspect of life, let alone in sport rehab and performance. Sharing clients and collaborating with other disciplines is a sign of strength. This allows us to focus on what we are good at; the athlete can benefit from everyone's expertise.

This is the heart of the modern athlete-centered model.

Everyone, including a doctor, chiropractor, physical therapist, athletic trainer, massage therapist, personal trainer, strength coach, and others, can offer insight to help an athlete achieve rehab and performance goals.

The following professional descriptions, based on the sequence an injured athlete might be treated, are not all-inclusive. If a specialty is not included in the list, it is not due to the lack of importance in the bridging-the-gap process. It is only due to the ever-growing number and types of professionals an athlete may encounter on the road to recovery.

### Medical Doctor (MD)—

Prior to practicing, MDs typically receive a four-year undergraduate education and four years of medical school, plus three to seven years of residency training, depending on the specialty. Many MDs complete fellowship training in specific areas following the residency.

An MD will assign a diagnosis based on tests performed, prescribe medication if needed, and, depending on the MD and the injury, might perform a needed surgery. The MD will work closely with the rehab team when progressing an athlete through rehab and then back to performance.

### Doctor of Osteopathy (DO)—

A DO has the same medical training and requirements as an MD. In addition to medical training, DOs learn osteopathic manual medicine and focus on holistic patient care.

### Physical Therapist (PT)—

Physical therapy education has changed in recent years. Currently, a PT will complete four years of undergraduate school and three years of PT school, entering the workforce with an entry-level doctorate (DPT).

A PT will examine a patient and treat to help decrease pain and improve movement and function. A PT can function in many specialty areas, such as pediatrics, cardiology, neurology, or orthopedics.

A sports PT has additional training working with athletes either by way of experience and taking the Sports Certified Specialist (SCS), being dual credentialed (AT/PT), or having completed a sports residency. All 50 states have some level of direct access to physical therapy; patients no longer have to see an MD prior to seeking treatment from a PT.

### Athletic Trainer (AT or ATC)—

Athletic trainers are multi-skilled health care professionals who collaborate with physicians to provide preventative services, emergency care, clinical diagnoses, therapeutic intervention, and rehabilitation of injuries and medical conditions.

Athletic trainers work under the direction of a physician as prescribed by state licensure statutes.[1] The current entry point into the profession of athletic training is a bachelor's degree; however, it was recently decided that the entry-level degree would be a master's, a change to be implemented by 2022.

### Chiropractor (DC)—

Chiropractors focus on musculoskeletal and nervous system issues, often treating neuromusculoskeletal disorders of the neck and back; however, DCs treat extremities and headache issues as well.

Chiropractors typically attend undergraduate school for four years, followed by four years of chiropractic-specific education focusing on manual therapy and adjustment techniques.

### Performance Specialist or Strength Coach—

There is a wide variety of paths to take to become a strength or performance coach. Most strength and performance coaches have a four-year undergraduate degree focusing on kinesiology or exercise science.

After this training, they often do a graduate assistantship, depending on the position desired. Passing a national exam is usually part of the process, such as Certified Strength and Conditioning Specialist (CSCS) or Strength and Conditioning Coach Certified (SCCC), among others.

### Skills Coach—

Skills coaches, such as pitching or defensive end coaches, may not have formal education in a specific area, but they are typically experts in the sport or position, often being athletes themselves.

They are an integral part of the return-to-play continuum and are the subject matter experts we turn to as part of our success with injured athletes. These coaches speak the language of the sport and often have great insight into the attributes needed for a successful return-to-play program.

An athlete might encounter many other professionals, including massage therapists, acupuncturists, nutritionists, and more. Consider where your skill set fits with the expertise of the other specialists in your care continuum, and recognize that there is a time and place for everyone to apply their knowledge.

Regardless of who is quarterbacking the care at the time, we focus on one thing above all: improving the athlete's health.

## WHO GUIDES THE PROCESS?

Where a client rests along the performance-training continuum will dictate the quarterback of that person's care at a given time. Ideally, someone different is in charge at each stage, depending on where the athlete is in this process.

When an athlete is injured during competition, the AT is the quarterback, determining vitals and the safety of the athlete's life and limbs. The AT determines if an athlete can safely return to play, or if immediate medical care is needed on the field.

If necessary, the AT determines how to safely remove the player from the field, performs or assists in assessments once off the field, and makes the needed referrals for quick diagnostics to determine the type and severity of the injury.

If the patient is post-operative, the doctor might be the quarterback, dictating precautions and contraindications after the surgery. As the rehab process moves on, a PT may take the lead, assisting the athlete in restoring the fundamentals of strength, range of motion, and proprioception.

When the client is ready to incorporate different training movements at various loads and speeds, a performance coach might take over. Finally, as the person begins to work on the technical and tactical aspects of the sport, a skills coach can play a lead role in re-familiarizing the athlete with the unique specifics of the sport or position.

There are obvious overlaps in these roles and the above descriptions are not dogmatic. Each team or situation has its unique way in which people work together to move this process along.

There is no single person who can do everything for an injured athlete, from on-the-field care, to post-injury evaluation, to the operating room, to skill and technique work at the practice facility, and all the steps between. We each need to be comfortable in the understanding that there are many contributors involved in the process, with certain people wearing larger hats at various times.

In the athlete-centered model, everyone has the athlete's best interest in mind. "Leave your letters at the door" was a common phrase for us EXOS, where I spent 13 years earlier in my career. The athlete is center stage at all times, no matter what the needs are at any point in time.

There is no room for ego in the athlete-centered model. There is too much to do, too much to work on and too much at stake for professionals to be arguing over who is in charge. We must be able to work together to return an athlete to the field, not only fully rehabbed, but hopefully as a stronger, healthier person.

Traditionally, the overall wellbeing of the athlete was not the focal point. Rehabilitation used to be concentrated on the isolated issue and its localized treatment. If an athlete was experiencing knee pain, this led the team's specialists to focus on evaluating the knee.

Treatment was directed at removing or reducing pain via local modalities or manual techniques. The athlete was given exercises to strengthen the surrounding muscles, or if the issue was more serious, surgery was performed and rehab commenced to return the athlete to pain-free function.

This model falls short when we look at individual specialists' actions and the sum total of these efforts. The main problem with this isolated, localized treatment approach is that it targets the supposed "source" of pain and related issues, such as swelling at the joint.

This is not the same as seeking to identify the *cause* of pain, such as faulty mechanics, neurological deficits, or an underlying structural issue.

Chasing pain, which is at best a lagging indicator of a problem, fails to see the person's entire kinetic chain and neuromusculoskeletal being, either in evaluation or during treatment. Thus, major gaps develop between the various steps needed to move from assessing an injury, rehabilitating an athlete, and returning the person to a game day–ready state.

A more comprehensive approach will accurately pinpoint the root of an injury so we can take the necessary corrective action to get the person back to play with sustainable motor patterns at the same or even a higher level than before the injury.

Evaluating injured tissues and joints, exploring kinetic linking and kinematic sequencing, and prescribing the appropriate solutions to return the athlete to full, healthy function cannot be done if we are only focusing on pain.

It also cannot be achieved if the specialists in the care continuum are working in isolation or fighting for control over the athlete's health and not communicating with others involved in the process.

The goal of helping athletes perform sustainably at their best for as long as possible is not achievable until we bridge the gap between rehabilitation and performance that plagues every level of every sport in which athletes get injured.

## STRUCTURE VERSUS FUNCTION

The word "function" is widely used in today's rehab and performance models. Functional exercises, functional evaluation, and functional progressions are just some of the ways we use this word when describing our examination or treatment philosophies.

What happened to structure? Does not anatomical structure dictate function?[2]

For example, if an athlete's femoral head and neck are rotated too far forward or too far backward—femoral anteversion or retroversion—as it relates to the femoral shaft, the person will have a difficult time squatting with the toes pointed forward.

The physical structure of the hip will prevent what most consider a neutral lower-extremity squat position, thus dictating the way the hip functions during a squat. We cannot go beyond the parameters of a body's structure.

With this same structure in a soccer player who is running, kicking, twisting, and turning during a game, the femoral head may be butting up against the acetabulum.

Thanks to Wolff's Law, we know if we do this enough, we will begin to change the structure, creating a cam or pincer lesion that might become problematic and hinder movement.[3] The function of repeated motion has changed the structure, which will in turn affect function in the weight room, on the pitch, or in daily activities.

We cannot look at function with blinders—we must consider structure, its influence on function, and reflect on how function can influence structure. This is a concept we will explore throughout this book.

Both structure and function need to be acknowledged and respected when examining a patient and creating a rehab program tailored to the person's specific needs.

As clinicians and strength coaches, we are comfortable with the musculoskeletal system. However, it is actually the *neuro*musculoskeletal system we are dealing with in our athletes. The nervous system and its central, autonomic, and peripheral subsets are what dictates musculoskeletal function.

Input dictates output. Bad input yields bad output. When we are not receiving quality information from visual, proprioceptive, and vestibular inputs, the data sent to the brain's movement centers and the motor output sent to the limbs will be suboptimal.

If we begin a movement from a structurally inadequate or inefficient position, the movement from that point forward will be inefficient.

However, we also need to define what an "inefficient movement pattern" really is. Often in the weight room or in training, we expect people to have "perfect form," our definition of what perfect form should be for that particular movement pattern.

Yet, the concept of "perfect movement" is arbitrary. What is perfect for you might not be perfect for me because of numerous factors, including our structural differences. If your client has what you consider a compensatory movement pattern, but has had that pattern for a long time, it is probably efficient energy expenditure and neural programming for that person.

If we change the compensatory movement pattern to what we believe is "better," we have increased the demands on the nervous system, as it needs to not only create new neural pathways to perform this movement, but also to destroy old neural pathways that allowed the movement to become almost reflexive.

We have also increased the metabolic demands on the system, making the new movement pattern more inefficient than the old pattern. As coaches, our concept of and desire for "proper movement" we want athletes to perform can actually make them less efficient in that movement pattern. We will discuss this more in the chapter on somatosensory control, beginning on page 123.

Prolonged posture or positioning will eventually dictate structure. Picture an older woman shuffling along a street. She may be overly kyphotic and seemingly unable to straighten her spine. This is not the result of a sudden trauma. Years of sitting, poor posture, and gravity have led to a permanent change in the spinal structure, creating the wedged vertebral bodies, degenerating discs, smaller foramen, and shortened soft tissue associated with this change in posture.

Changing the structure or function of a degenerated spinal column will be difficult once these anatomical changes occur—perhaps impossible—although there is hope, using movement skills both ancient and new.

We cannot separate structure and function. This is why *Structure & Function* is the name of my education company. These two independent things are interdependent upon one another.

## THE ORGANIZATIONAL SYSTEM SLIDE

Phil Sizer and I met in 2007 when I was on a quest to return to my physical therapy roots after living for years in the performance world. Phil is a lead instructor for the International Academy of Orthopedic Medicine–United States (IAOM–US) and is a professor at Texas Tech University. In contrast to me, he had been living in the PT world for decades at the time and was moving toward the performance realm. We are both PTs, coming at an organizational system from opposite sides.

Our early discussion brought us to what we fondly called "The Slide" when we were creating a master diagram for a presentation. The slide was a representation of hours upon hours of discussion, debate, and research. It became my organizational system and is now how I teach the model of bridging the gap from rehab to performance.

The slide references structure and function, as well as the clinical and performance aspects of return to play. It acknowledges the biopsychosocial factors that serve as the foundation of individual responses and tolerance. It reminds us that everything—every philosophy, every school of thought, every letter we have after our names—has its place in returning an athlete to a sport.

We just need to understand how and where things fit together, and how to sequence them.

**Figure 1.1—The Slide**

*The Slide is the organizational framework Phil Sizer and I developed in 2008 to help organize the concepts of Bridging the Gap from Rehab to Performance. It has framed and shaped my approach to rehab ever since.*

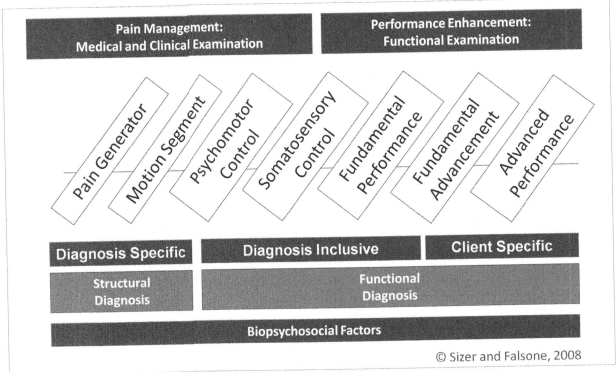

© Sizer and Falsone, 2008

First, we need to recognize there are both clinical and performance perspectives. That does not necessarily mean these are different or that we need to discuss them in a different manner.

However, perspective can change reality and we need to understand that there are different viewpoints represented in the rehab-to-performance model.

Once an athlete is injured, we develop a clinical diagnosis, such as rotator cuff tendonitis, as well as a functional diagnosis like scapular dyskinesis, and then use both to guide the athlete's journey back to full health.

Indeed, many different clinical diagnoses may share the same functional diagnosis.

When someone is in pain, we need to address the symptom. Even though we do not always follow pain or focus solely on its alleviation, there are many studies that demonstrate that function is altered in the presence of pain.[4,5,6,7]

We cannot ignore pain and simply perform "functional" activities. When either acute or chronic pain is present, we are in the medical model of patient care. It is only after the person is out of pain that we can move to a more performance-oriented model of athlete care.

In the medical model, we do typical diagnostic tests and clinical examinations. When someone is at the medical-focused end of the spectrum, we need diagnostic tests and clinical exams. These might be required to document progress and ensure proper

tissue healing has occurred and that it will continue.

Later, in the performance model, we can conduct our functional evaluations. Some functional testing might be appropriate in the medical aspect of the spectrum. However, pain might give us false information in that testing, and that should instead be done when the athlete is no longer in pain.

## PAIN MANAGEMENT: MEDICAL AND CLINICAL EXAMINATION

When we are in pain, everything is different. Movement patterns are often altered.[8] Anxiety, depression, stress, and fear are common.[9]

Making the correct diagnosis early is paramount in order to place the person on the proper rehabilitation path. There are two types of diagnoses we need to properly rehabilitate an athlete in pain.

The first is a structural diagnosis. A medical or clinical exam may include clinical tests such as X-rays or MRIs and a structural injury might be confirmed. A torn ligament, fractured bone, or degenerative tendon is may be diagnosed as the tissue with the problem. Surgery is often an option in this phase.

## PERFORMANCE ENHANCEMENT: FUNCTIONAL EXAMINATION

A functional diagnosis is the second type of needed diagnosis.[10] A functional diagnosis typically describes a reason or cause for pain versus injured tissue, which might be the source of the pain.

An example of a functional diagnosis might be scapular dyskinesis, a scapula that is not well controlled or moving correctly. Scapular dyskinesia may be the reason for shoulder impingement and an inflamed tendon, and the inflamed tendon is the structural issue related to the movement problem.

A functional diagnosis is more about movement issues and deficiencies versus structural anomalies and pathologies.

## DIAGNOSIS-SPECIFIC

In the diagnosis-specific segment, the treatment interventions are exactly that—diagnosis-specific, meaning it matters if the athlete has a herniated disk or spinal stenosis. We might perform two very different immediate treatment interventions based on a diagnosis.

For example, if someone has a shoulder bursitis, cross-friction massage may irritate the inflamed bursae and make the pain worse.

However, if the person has a chronic shoulder tendinosis, cross-friction massage may significantly help.

We base acute treatment interventions upon the pathological tissue, the normal tissue-healing properties of that tissue, and account for how that tissue will physiologically respond to the selected intervention.

The treatment is likely dictated by the structural diagnosis made during the clinical examination.

## DIAGNOSIS-INCLUSIVE

From a treatment standpoint, a diagnosis-inclusive treatment is performed regardless of which tissue is the problem. For example, if someone has a herniated disk in the low back, a spondylolisthesis, or spinal stenosis, it does not matter at this stage.

Here, everyone will get some type of core stability activities. If one person has a posterior impingement at the shoulder or another has had a shoulder subluxation, they will both get some type of scapular-controlled mobility and rotator cuff exercises.

In this phase, the diagnosis does not specifically affect the treatment, which is most likely done to address the functional diagnosis made during the performance exam.

## CLIENT-SPECIFIC

Finally, during the rehab process it matters if we are dealing with a baseball player, a football player, or a computer engineer who runs marathons on occasional weekends. All three athletes need to run, but they all run differently.

A baseball player needs acceleration and absolute speed mechanics in a specific direction, taking into account hitting a thick base at given intervals, as well as deceleration.

The football player who is an offensive lineman needs acceleration mechanics, but may not need absolute speed, as offensive linemen typically do not run that far. A receiver will most certainly need acceleration, absolute speed, and deceleration, along with vestibular considerations, as receivers are often looking in directions other than where they are moving. Finally, the marathon runner does not need acceleration mechanics, although this could be argued, but certainly needs absolute speed mechanics.

All three of these scenarios require running, but running in a specific manner for the sport or position. Our interventions need to be client-specific based on the goals for rehab.

## THE SEGMENTS OF THE ORGANIZATIONAL SYSTEM

Now that we have covered some of the basic principles that form the foundation of the organizational system, let us take a closer look at its segments, each of which has its own chapter for further exploration.

This is not a dogmatic classification system. Many interventions or schools of thought might fall into more than one category. Each intervention has many parts to it, and in your thought process, one might fit into an entirely different category than listed in this book. This is fine. As you work through the chapters and begin to understand the system, think about where each of the phases, disciplines, and concepts fit into your personal practice.

All models fit, all disciplines fit, and all "gurus" fit when we work to bridge the gap between rehabilitation and performance. Whatever your specialty, decide where that school of thought lies in this system as you create a process to return athletes to sports performance.

We will look at an overview of each category next, and expand upon them in individual chapters.

Briefly, think about when a client comes to you in pain. Say, for example, the person is a soccer player with a painful groin. First, we need to decide what tissue is the issue. We need to identify the *pain generator*.

Is the pain coming from a torn muscle or tendon in the adductors or in the abdomen? Is the pain coming from the hip-joint capsule impinged between two bones? Is the pain coming from a degenerated joint surface?

Are all structures of the hip normal and the pain is coming from the low back or the central nervous system?

Once this is determined, we need to ensure the joint is moving properly in relation to those around it. Does the hip have full range of motion? Is flexibility normal? Are all aspects of the joint working well so it can fit within the system as part of a whole? Can the lumbar spine stabilize in order for the hip to move? Are there limitations at the ankle that could be affecting the hip? This section will take into account the entire *motion segment*.

We then need to make sure the right muscles are firing at the right time. We need to ensure there is proper *psychomotor control*. Is the glute acting as a prime mover for hip extension, or are the hamstrings or lumbarparaspinals dominating the movement pattern?

From here, we move into *somatosensory control*. We consider all aspects of the neurological system—including reflexes, visual, vestibular—and all the neuromotor programming elements affecting how the motion segment moves or why pain is being generated. This is the largest and most complicated category and certainly influences and is influenced by every other aspect.

Next, we have *fundamental performance*. Not only does the hip itself have foundational strength—which could also fall under the motion-segment category—but we look to see that the entire system has proper fundamental strength to be expressed as power in our next category, *fundamental advancement*.

It is within fundamental advancement that we begin to move at various loads and speeds, introducing fundamental athletic movements such as acceleration, crossover, drop step, and more.

Finally, in *advanced performance*, we begin to meet the client-specific goals of returning to an activity. Whether the client is a hockey player, lacrosse player, or laborer, we introduce the specific movement requirements that must be mastered prior to returning to the activity.

Of course, underlying this whole strategy are the *biopsychosocial* factors that influence how we each have a different response to pain and to the planned and executed interventions.

The biochemical, nutritional, and genetic factors of each person's biology will affect the mindset, mood, and attitude of the person.

The societal, familial, and cultural influences on a person will impact how that person responds to any stimulus.

The biopsychosocial influencers are the individual factors we must consider every time; they will never be the same for any two people.

No single part of the continuum is necessarily a prerequisite to another. Many of these areas can and should be addressed simultaneously as an athlete progresses from table to field. However, these all need to be considered prior to an athlete successfully returning to play.

## Pain Generator

In Chapter Two, the section on determining the pain generator, we identify the problem tissue. It matters whether we are dealing with a bursa or a tendon.

If the client is struggling to manage a bursitis and we attempt tool-assisted soft-tissue work on the inflamed bursa, we might make things worse. However, if we are dealing with a tendinopathy, soft-tissue treatment might significantly help the healing process.

In another case, if the athlete has disc-originating pain, trunk flexion might exacerbate the symptoms. If we are instead looking at a stenosis, trunk flexion might improve the symptoms. Accurately identifying the problem tissue is important for us to appropriately direct our initial treatment efforts.

If you do not have examinations and assessments in your toolbox, befriend a diagnostician and share patients and clients with that person. You do not need to learn how to assess, but you do need to understand assessment and have a referral policy in place.

If no pain generator is present—such as in a patient with phantom-limb pain, chronic pain, or non-specific lower-back pain (NSLBP)—we need to use other identifiers, such as restricted range of motion, compromised movement patterns, a lack of stability, neurological influences, or biopsychosocial considerations to guide us to the area that needs our first attention.

Someone who is in pain without the presence of a pain generator presents a challenging situation. There is no nociceptive stimulation to alter; therefore, our typical pain-eliminating techniques will not work.

In the initial pain discovery, we are defining which "tissue is the issue." As an example, in my case, I might draw from my manual therapy and differential diagnosis background to determine the problem at hand.

To determine a working diagnosis for the patient in front of me, this might involve applying the skills learned in physical therapy or athletic training schools or things I mastered when studying for my certification in orthopedic manual therapy.

We might be concerned about pain and want to decrease it by using a method such as kinesiology tape.[11] Perhaps other standard modalities will assist in pain reduction. There are many clinical interventions to choose from; your list of skills will be different, and that will guide your choices.

## Motion Segment

We need to reestablish the proper use of the entire motion segment, and not just a localized injury site or the source of pain. For example, if we are dealing with an elbow issue, we need to make sure the cervical spine, shoulder complex, elbow, wrist, and hand are all working as a unit—this is the focus of Chapter Four.

We should also ensure that there has not been loss of compensatory range of motion elsewhere in the body.

The nervous system prioritizes protection of painful tissue, and adjusts movement accordingly.[12] Through proper neuromusculoskeletal evaluation, the diagnostician will be able to determine if and where the body has compensated to protect the injured tissue.

I once had an athlete who had dislocated his elbow in a traumatic manner. Despite our good efforts, he ended up with a shoulder issue, including loss of motion and pain because he was guarded and afraid to move his arm away from his body. As a result, dysfunction developed in the segment next to the injury site, which in this case was the shoulder.

We may not be able to prevent everything, but we know that the motion segments that make up and surround an injured limb or the spinal segments above and below an injury can become compromised due to fear, avoidance, and pain.[13,14]

There could also be a restriction along a fascial line feeding tension upstream, downstream, or both.[15] You can define a motion segment in many ways. You could simply consider an upper extremity, spine, or lower extremity as the motion segment, or you could think of it even broader than that, following fascial lines or kinetic chains.

However you define the motion segment for a given patient, you must address and consider it throughout the rehabilitative process, rather than just looking at a joint or tissue in isolation.

Bring the concepts of biotensegrity to mind when thinking of motion segments. Biotensegrity applies the mathematical concept of tensegrity to the human body.[16] Tensegrity, developed by R. Buckminster Fuller between the 1920s and 1940s, is the concept that a three-dimensional structure is under constant tension with intermittent periods of compression to maintain the structure's stability.

Biotensegrity states that in the human body, all levels—including molecular, cellular, tissue, organ, and organ systems—are operating in the same manner.

Humans will maintain their general form despite gravity because of the constant state of tension with intermittent compression that occurs throughout the body. Our bodily systems, down to the molecular level, are built upon this constant tension.

Our movement choices and postures will introduce the necessary compressive forces to allow the body to change and adapt, all while maintaining the general human form.

When we think of the body as a tensegrity system, we realize we never do movement in isolation. In order for movement in one area to occur, a resultant compression or tension must occur elsewhere to allow that to happen. This concept demonstrates a system in which nothing occurs in isolation.

While we consider these concepts and interventions, we are concerned with how the client is or is not using the entire affected limb.

We might pull from manual therapy, mobilization with movement, or tool-assisted soft-tissue work to reestablish the motion-segment function. Dry needling or cupping might be a suitable intervention choice. Alternatively, we might perhaps use fascial or visceral manipulation to deal with the affected area.

Corrective exercises learned during the Functional Movement Screen (FMS®), the Selective Functional Movement Assessment (SFMA®), or Functional Range Conditioning® (FRC) training could come in handy. Muscle activation techniques (MAT™) might also be applicable in this stage as we try to get the entire limb and motion segment functioning normally.

The options in this phase are almost limitless, based on your training and area of focus.

## Psychomotor Control

In reviewing psychomotor control, which we will do in Chapter Five, we are concerned with the appropriate tissue firing at the right time as muscles and other tissues do their jobs. Prime movers must remain prime movers. Synergists must be synergists, and stabilizers must be stabilizers.

When a stabilizer such as lumbar musculature becomes a synergist to hip extension, or a synergist like the hamstrings becomes a prime mover, or a prime mover like a glute decreases its activity because another muscle is doing its job, the body gets angry and it will produce pain.

Just as in a factory, the body has individual parts responsible for a job. When people in a factory start doing jobs they were not intended to do, the entire line gets thrown off. One job has too many workers, while another has no one focusing on it. Chaos ensues, and in our example, pain is created in the body.

Neuromuscular control of the body is the fine-tuning we use to ensure proper movement. Of course, the body will figure things out if needed and will compensate its way through a less-than-ideal motor pattern.[17] That newly created motor pattern certainly has the potential to be efficient; however,

biomechanical stresses caused during these compensations can cause damage if left unattended.

Over time, this compensation can lead to pain or asymmetries in flexibility and strength, and will further exacerbate the issue. The compensatory pattern will become the default pattern once the brain myelinates this new workaround.

There are many schools of thought in psychomotor control to pull from, including Dynamic Neuromuscular Stabilization® (DNS), Postural Restoration Institute® (PRI), MAT, dry needling, FMS, SFMA, Shirley Saharmann's work in Movement System Impairments, and Pilates, to name a few. We use whatever aligns best with our specific training and practice.

## Biopsychosocial Considerations

The biopsychosocial model was introduced in 1977 by psychiatrist George Engel.[18] In this model, he suggests that the person's biology, psychology, and social aspects of life have an influence on each other and the human as a whole being. These three things in combination will dictate pain, suffering, and response to treatment interventions, and this is what we discuss in Chapter Six.

The psychological stress of an injury can increase stress hormones and inflammatory markers, making a somatic injury difficult to heal. Social activities such as drinking and smoking all impact a person's overall health and wellbeing.

Lack of support from family and friends can increase depression, impacting a person's biology. It can also lead to unhealthy lifestyle behaviors such as substance abuse, interrupted sleep, or poor eating habits, thereby impacting the biological ability to heal.

In fact, biopsychosocial factors could be argued as the number-one element that will impact your patients' ability to heal and return to play.

We have all had experiences when we had two people who play the same sport walk in the door with the same diagnosis, and later have two very different outcomes. Biopsychosocial factors that are individual to each person are most likely at play when that happens.

When dealing with any athlete, we must recognize that the injury impacts the psychological wellbeing of that person. How someone deals with the trauma will be dictated by social support and techniques used to cope with the stresses of injury. These stresses will impact biology and the person's ability to heal.

We cannot ignore these factors in this work as we are bridging the gap from rehab to performance.

## Somatosensory Control

The somatosensory system, covered in Chapter Seven, is a system of nerve receptors and cells that sense and react to alterations in a body's internal state. We could not have a motor system without a sensory system. Our input gives us our output. Bad input equals bad output.

If we continually type the wrong command into a computer keyboard, we keep getting the wrong output. We have to give the computer the correct commands for it to work properly.

The same goes for our bodies. If we send faulty information, our motor responses will be wrong and potentially inefficient. When we are dealing with somatosensory control,[19] we are addressing vestibular balance, postural sway, reflexes, visual system, and proprioceptive awareness.[20]

This phase of moving from rehabilitation to performance centers on reestablishing balance and postural reflexes and creating better sensory input for improved motor output.[21] Here, concepts of motor learning and motor control are of use, and we might apply techniques from DNS, PRI, yoga or Pilates to assist the client with balance, proprioception, and reflexive responses.

## Fundamental Performance

As we start to look toward performance, which we will do in Chapter Nine, we begin to address fundamental strength. Does each muscle have the basic foundational strength to carry out the task we are asking it to do? Does each muscle have the ability to fire, against gravity, with resistance?

During standardized manual muscle testing, does each muscle possess the ability to perform at a foundational "five out of five" strength—the normal muscle strength per manual muscle testing principles?[22,23]

If not, we have some basic strength training work to do. We cannot build power—the forceful application of strength—without first building baseline strength. In this stage, we need to reestablish fundamental strength and ultimately power.

Deploying foundational corrective exercises for strength will work well during this phase. Correctives derived from FMS, SFMA, PRI, MAT, and strength and conditioning training are used to produce the strength needed to prepare for more powerful movements.

When introducing power, it does not matter whether this is from a kettlebell, Olympic lifting, or another approach. Use whatever you think will work best for a client, given the medical history, sports background, training age, and performance needs.

## Fundamental Advancement

During the fundamental-advancement phase, Chapter Ten, we study how to display foundational strength—fundamental performance—as an expression of power, and apply this power to general athletic movement. This is the phase where we introduce power production and focus on linear movement, multi-directional movement, jumping, and landing.

For example, an athlete must be able to achieve the fundamental positions needed for acceleration before we program sprints. Athletes need to be able to manage the forces created during the acceleration and then be able to safely decelerate to avoid injury.

During this progression of bridging the gap, a recovering athlete must relearn proper backpedaling, shuffling, jumping, landing, and basic footwork techniques before returning to full practices and games.[24] These fundamental athletic skills are required in every athlete, in different combinations, and at various loads and speeds. This is the time to rebuild the foundation of athletic movement.

The primary goal at this point is to retrain universal athletic movements and power creation and management. This is when we use the skills from the strength and conditioning models. It is up to you whether you follow principles employed by EXOS, Michael Boyle, Dan John, standard CSCS formulas, or any other approach.

Attention to your individual client's needs based on the medical history, the sport, and your experience will serve your client well.

## Advanced Performance

Once we get to performance, which we will do in Chapter Eleven, the unique requirements of each sport and the different positions start to come into play. For example, whether a football player is a wide receiver or an offensive lineman, both athletes need to run, but an offensive lineman most likely needs acceleration mechanics more than absolute speed mechanics.

Consider a baseball and a soccer player: The former needs to run around the bases and to various fielding positions while paying attention to where a ball is as it flies through the air, while the latter must run down and across the pitch with a ball at foot, avoiding opponents along the way. Although these athletes share fundamental athletic movements, each sport and each position within a sport have different needs from a movement perspective, and we address those needs in a slightly different way.

This brings us to a fundamental concept when organizing an intervention: *Are we offering something to the athlete that is diagnosis-specific, diagnosis-inclusive, or client-specific?*

Our treatments in the pain generator and motion segments are typically based on the diagnosis—these are *diagnosis-specific.* In the early rehab phase, it is important to know whether we are dealing with a bursitis or tendonitis, and it matters how that pain generator is affecting the entire limb or motion segment.

As we move forward through rehabilitation, the interventions become *diagnosis-inclusive.* This means that most likely we will prescribe some form of "core stability" work to everyone in the facility—however we choose to define that core stability.

The 60-year-old golfer gets a set of core stability exercises, as does the 14-year-old high school football player and the 24-year-old professional athlete.[25] These are different age populations with different performance goals and, probably, different diagnoses, but they all need some type of "core stability" to improve the conditions.

Finally, as we work our way toward the more performance-centric end of the bridging-the-gap model, we must be more *client-specific.*

The firefighter and the professional athlete will both need to function at a very high level, but they will do it in different ways. The quarterback and the pitcher may both be professional athletes, but their jobs require different skills. We need to consider the individual needs of the athletes in order to restore full function and return them to their sports.[26]

This performance phase aims to return the client to the sport, with position-specific functions needed for that sport and position. As with the rehabilitation interventions, it does not matter which performance model you choose. These are your personal preferences and prerogative as a practitioner or coach.

Be sure to include skills coaches in this segment, as it is essential to enable the client to meet the unique technical demands of the sport and position.

You can also apply the kind of movement analysis used at EXOS, described beginning on page 238, to ensure the client has regained full capacity in each of the main movement patterns needed to retake the field.

## SHIFTING BETWEEN A MEDICAL AND A PERFORMANCE MODEL

This is one of the most difficult concepts to capture in a book. There is no single defining point where an athlete is doing rehab and then making the transition to performance training. Our athletes may rehabbing an upper-extremity injury, and at the same time be performing lower-body performance training to minimize atrophy and maintain the ability to produce power in the legs while still protecting the injury.

Although the bridging-the-gap model seems like a continuum, it is actually more of a checklist. Your athletes do not need to pass one stage before moving to the next. These elements do not have to happen in a certain order, with the exception of addressing the pain generator, if there is one.

Pain will affect all aspects of the bio-psychosocial model, which is covered in Chapter Six, and needs to be dealt with immediately. With that exception, everything else may be worked on at any point in the process of returning to play, but these all need to be addressed at some point prior to returning an injured athlete to the field.

However, there are plenty of athletes playing while in pain. While the bridging-the-gap model acknowledges that pain should be dealt with immediately, this idealistic suggestion may not be a realistic expression of what occurs every day in sport.

People participate while they are in pain—they do it all the time. Hence, this model is not a true continuum, but more of an ideal, theoretical progression that recognizes the need for flexibility toward a given athlete at a given time.

The first four categories of *Pain Generator, Motion Segment, Psychomotor Control,* and *Somatosensory Control* live under the medical model. We typically address these areas under the supervision of a health care provider with a focus on improving

pain, normalizing a system, and preparing for the higher-level activities of the performance model. These four areas deal with the fundamental building blocks of performance.

*Somatosensory Control, Fundamental Performance, Fundamental Advancement,* and *Advanced Performance* are part of the performance model. These typically build and fine-tune an athletic body after laying the foundation.

The overlap of the two models comes from the nervous systems. Somatosensory control—the afferent nervous system—is the underlying key to everything. It will be difficult to build total-body strength and power, athletic movement, and athletic skill in a person who is in pain, lacks proper mobility and stability, and has poor body control.

Athletes always want to be in the performance model. Athletes will come to you with goals such as "I want to improve my first-step quickness," yet have horrible hip mobility and cannot get into the fundamental athletic positions needed to improve first-step quickness.

Restoring the motion segment might be necessary in the immediate stages of intervention. Once the motion segment is improved, first-step quickness improves because you have addressed the weakest link in the system.

Philosophies and techniques that are more on the medical model side of the continuum should improve the performance model without doing anything related to performance.

Think of the medical model as the foundation for a new house, and the performance model as the actual house to be built upon that foundation. Can you build a house on a bad foundation? Of course you can.

However, you will be limited as to how many stories the house can have, how big the house can be, and how long the house will be able to withstand the elements. You can build a house on a bad foundation, but it is not advisable.

Likewise, building performance on an injured, broken system is possible, but it is not advisable.

## CREATING A RETURN-TO-PLAY TIMELINE

People in our fields often work without a plan. Could you imagine getting on a flight and having the pilot not follow the preflight checklist and executing the flight plan? Alternatively, imagine trying to build a house without a blueprint. Plans direct us where to go. They force us to go through the systematic processes to ensure we do not skip a fundamental step that may be impossible to fix later.

Creating long-term goals with short-term milestones to be met along the way will ensure that you give your client ample time to adapt, and these allow everyone to see the roadmap they will be traveling along. If anything veers off course, the end result will change.

Let us use a soccer player returning to the field after a knee injury, whom we would like to have back on the field in a game in three months.

We need to look at the schedule and see if there is time to set up a simulated or friendly game that may not have much at stake. We aim for some type of lower-intensity, full game activity one week prior to the athlete's real return to see how well the action of a simulated game is tolerated.

Once we determine the day, we know to plan short games first, playing with a full team of 11 on each side, but with a shortened field so there is less running for our returning player. We might want that to happen one or two weeks prior to a full pitch simulated game.

Prior to that, we could schedule a game with shorter distances on the pitch, with fewer players on the field to focus more on offensive or defensive plays. We want that to happen a week prior to playing with a full team on each side.

Earlier, we would plan offensive or defensive drills with some light contact, and before that, drills without the possibility of contact. Before that, we would have used drills that do not require critical thinking—just movement execution—and before that, we would use multi-directional movement skills specific to soccer, while using a ball.

Before that, the athlete needs multi-directional movement skills specific to soccer, but without a ball. Prior to that, we would plan linear movement, with and without a ball.

Before performing linear movement, we need to see full strength and the ability to develop power.

In order to do this, an athlete needs full mobility and stability throughout the motion segment, with good psychomotor control and somatosensory control.

Prior to this, our athlete needs to be free of pain. By the time you work backward through that entire scenario, giving the athlete plenty of time to adapt to the new stresses, you may find that three months is not enough time to return the person to play.

If you were to attempt it, the progressions would have to be extremely aggressive and there would be no room for issues in the process.

If there is an increase in pain or swelling at any point, you would need to take a step backward, and the long-term goal of returning to the field would be delayed.

Reaching your short-term goals will culminate in achieving your long-term goal. You cannot achieve long-term aims without covering the short-term ones along the way.

From a clinical standpoint, we have to make our findings and explanation of dysfunctions meaningful. When we are evaluating a patient and decide we see a weak glute medius…truly, who cares? Why should anyone care that the glute med is weak?

Well, a weak glute med will lead to poor hip mechanics, possibly resulting in synergistic dominance of the TFL and

decreased power production at the hip, overloading the lumbar spine or knee. Once we relate the objective dysfunction to a functional limitation, we can create a goal: improve glute med strength. Once we have a goal, we can create a plan. The plan should include glute med strengthening exercises.

Every objective dysfunction should have a functional limitation along with a short-term or long-term goal, with a plan to achieve the goal.

To be sure, I always tie an objective dysfunction with meaningful information, which you will see in the chart found in Appendix Two. This keeps me honest in making sure every objective finding has a plan for improvement, as well as making sure every dysfunction is attached to a meaningful functional impairment.

Don't identify dysfunction for the sake of identifying dysfunction. What does the dysfunction mean? How does it affect the patient's life, and how are you going to fix it?

## CLINICAL PEARL

- Identify an objective dysfunction
- Attach it to a functional limitation
- Determine a short- or long-term goal for improvement
- Create a plan to fix it

Create realistic timelines for your athletes to adapt to the new stresses you are introducing, and build in some recovery days to allow for rest. Work backward from the long-term goal to give you, the athlete and the coach a realistic timeline for return to play.

## SUMMARY

Bridging the gap from rehab to performance does not follow a linear continuum. If we wait for all football players to have perfect fundamental performance and somatosensory control, we would all be staring at a blank television on Sundays. Nor are the sports medicine and sports-performance elements of athletic rehab going to represent a perfect sequence.

We might be working in several of these phases at the same time and might have to regress certain exercises to ensure quality movement patterns.[27] The organization of the bridging-the-gap model should help you and your team understand where each intervention fits, and this will not necessarily be a linear progression.

In a clinical and performance world where there are so many experts to follow, the development of a philosophical training model can be difficult to create and implement, especially for the less-experienced practitioner.

Rather than trying to be exclusive or exclusionary, remember that many schools of thought, when broken down to their core principles, all focus on the same thing. All techniques, exercise types, schools of thought, and training principles are valuable when bridging the gap from rehab to performance.

It is your job to figure out the best way to combine your education in the most effective and efficient ways possible to get your athletes back onto the field. I hope the material presented in this book will help you do exactly that. That is the beauty of this system.

You do not have to choose one person to follow nor do you need to adhere to a specific system. If it had been proven that a single system worked, we would all be doing it. Everything fits and has its place. Your choices are dependent upon the individual athlete in your care.

# CHAPTER TWO
## PAIN GENERATOR

When it comes to the rehabilitation phase of bridging the gap, we should not chase pain, nor should we consider it the only indicator of dysfunction. It should not be the only symptom we try to help alleviate. That is not to say that we can or should ignore pain, either.

Many people struggle with pain on a daily basis, and very few—old or young, recreational athletes, or pros, or anyone in between—can claim to be pain free.

Indeed, a 2015 study in the *Journal of Pain* found that 126.1 million people reported pain in the three months before the survey, and that was just those who held up their hands. Of these, 25.3 million said they had chronic pain, while 39.8 million reported pain at level of three or four, the kind that impacts overall health and wellbeing. Clearly, pain is a widespread problem.[28]

We break pain into two distinct categories: acute and chronic. Acute pain manifests itself quickly and often results directly from an identifiable injury. This type of pain typically responds to traditional interventions.

On the other hand, chronic pain is the kind that lasts for three or more months, does not respond to typical pain treatment methods, and is considered to be its own disease process rather than tied to an injury, even if an injury was the initial cause of the preceding acute pain.

It is the clinician's job help restore full motion in movement patterns, and also to help our clients be free of pain. This often coincides with improving mobility and eliminating other symptoms tied to the pain generator. As physical therapist and creator of MobilityWod Kelly Starrett says, "Painful tissue is dysfunctional tissue."

If we can eliminate the dysfunction, we also have a good shot at helping people get out of pain.

## PAIN THEORIES

As we try to understand why the body deals with pain the way it does and as we dive into the research, we discover some potentially conflicting theories to explain the mechanism of pain-generation pathways.

Pain involves many systems—the peripheral, central, and autonomic nervous systems, the structural-anatomical system, the limbic system, and the cardiovascular system, just to name a few.

There are still regions of the brain we do not understand, and we do not have a definitive, all-encompassing pain model that covers all the bases.

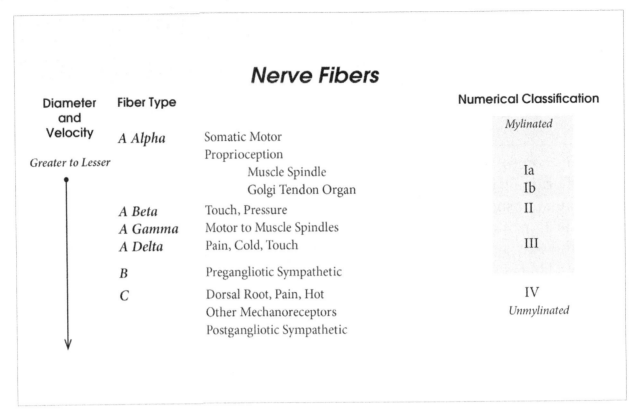

**Figure 2.1—Nerve Fibers**

*The body is made up of a vast network of afferent nerve fibers that bring information from the outside world to the central nervous system for interpretation. Nerve fibers are of varying diameters and have varying amounts of myelin, an insulating and protective sheath around the nerve.*

*Because of these differences in size and insulation, the velocity that information travels from the periphery to the central nervous system is different, depending on which afferent nerve is stimulated. This means information reaches the central nervous system at different times.*

Nonetheless, here is an overview of a few of the most popular theories.

## Specificity Theory

Max Von Frey developed one of the earliest theories of pain in 1895: the Specificity Theory. This theory states that individual pain receptors transmit signals to a specific pain center in the brain, which then sends back instructions for the appropriate motor response, such as to quickly pull a hand away from the hot pan.[29] This theory is based on the assumption that there is a specific pain system.

While the sheer simplicity of this notion is comforting, it has been disproven: There is no identifiable pain center in the brain. This theory also fails to acknowledge the psychological aspect of pain or the role that prior experience can have in making us hypersensitive to various pain stimuli.

## Pattern Theory

In the late 1920s and early 1930s, John Paul Nafe and Johannes Scheider suggested[30] that there is no distinct system for sensing and responding to pain, but that pain receptors are shared with other bodily systems.

In this theory, the brain only gets a pain signal if there is a specific combination and summation of stimuli formed in the spinal cord, which leads to the implementation of a preset pattern of responses.

One of the problems with the pattern theory is that it underestimates the role of the brain, viewing it merely as the receiver of a message from the receptors. We now know the brain plays a far more complicated and dynamic role in how the body deals with pain.

## Gate Control Theory

Next up in our pain study is the sensory theory, which operates on the idea of "gate control." The Gate Control Theory, developed in 1965 by Ronald Melzack and Patrick Wall, is the idea that when you slam a finger in a door, you would wrap the finger in the other hand or perhaps put it in your mouth, caress it, or do anything you can to relieve the pain.[31]

All peripheral sensations—heat, cold, touch, pain, vibration—are transmitted by peripheral nerve stimulation. This stimulation of nerves is transmitted to the spinal cord and, if significant enough, information is transmitted to the brain for processing.

Pain sensation is carried by nociceptive pain fibers, also known as A-Delta and C-Fibers. These signals go to the dorsal horn of the spinal cord, stimulate a second-order neuron, and then travel via the lateral spinothalamic tract to the brain for interpretation. If we add some form of touch to the equation, we also stimulate A-Beta fibers.

The touch sensation travels via A-Beta fibers to the spinal cord as well, stimulates an inhibitory interneuron in the dorsal horn, and diminishes the pain sensation that travels to the brain via the afferents stimulated by the A-Delta and C-Fibers. We feel "less" pain.

This, again, is why we are quick to squeeze or caress a finger after we shut it in a door—this actually diminishes the pain sensation perceived by the brain.

Gate Control Theory makes a lot of sense in many scenarios, but it does not explain those in which a nociceptor—the sensory receptors for pain—are not stimulated and yet a person still experiences pain.

## Conditioned Pain Modulation

The Conditioned Pain Modulation theory summarizes[32] what you might have experienced at the hand of an older sibling. You can probably remember when you were younger and crying because your arm hurt; your brother punched you in the other arm and said, "Do you feel better? Now you are not thinking about your hurt arm anymore."

That summarizes the Conditioned Pain Modulation theory, which states that pain inhibits pain. Two noxious stimuli are applied at the same time—the second in the same area, but not in the same spot as the first. The second stimulus is processed by the dorsal horn and can inhibit the first noxious stimuli.

This theory holds up, and may be why when we are applying a pain-reducing technique of any sort, simply being *near* the area can be as effective as being on the area.

## Neuromatrix of Pain

Other pain theories assign an important role to localized tissue and the peripheral nerves located at the site of the pain event. In contrast, The Neuromatrix of Pain view emphasizes the role of the brain, shifting focus to components of the central nervous system (CNS).[33]

In this theory, pain is actually the output of the brain; the multiple influences on pain outside of peripheral nociceptive stimulation are important.

The Neuromatrix of Pain emphasizes the brain's decision to create a pain sensation and diminishes the input from peripheral tissue. It does not negate the peripheral nervous system's part.

Peripheral noxious stimulation still plays a large role in the creation of a pain sensation, but it does not provide the entire story.

This theory does a much better job of explaining phantom-limb pain, fibromyalgia, NSLBP, and other chronic pain conditions where nociceptive

stimulation is not present, but the sensation of pain persists.

## THE MEANING OF PAIN

Lorimer Moseley is an influential person in pain theory, and I highly recommend his video, aptly named *Pain,* for an entertaining, simple overview of this highly complex topic. Moseley describes pain as holding meaning: It is personal.[34]

The pain I experience is not the pain you experience, even if we have similar nociceptive stimulation and the same diagnosis. Pain can be more psychological than physiological.

For example, say we were walking on a beach and both of us stepped on something sharp. While we would both wince, I might be able to continue our walk.

However, perhaps you had previously cut your foot and the cut became infected, which required a hospital stay and a two-week course of antibiotics. You might demand that I either carry you back to the car or go for help. It would be the same experience for both of us, but with a different frame of reference to interpret the stimulus of stepping on something sharp.

We need to be conscious when dealing with people having the same diagnosis because they could have very different pain perceptions. We cannot judge one person's pain based on the objective findings of a diagnosis.

Sometimes people might have a catastrophic injury and feel minimal pain, and yet another might have a minor hamstring strain and be limping in severe distress.

Pain is subjective. It is individual. We cannot assume that the same nociceptive stimulation in two people will result in the same perceived sensation or experience.

---

## CLINICAL PEARL

Pain is subjective, individual, cultural, situational, central, peripheral, conscious, and emotional.

It is always unpleasant and is associated with actual or potential tissue damage.[35]

---

## AN INJURY EVENT: THE TWO STAGES OF ACUTE PAIN

When we are injured, we often talk of how much something hurts, but that is an oversimplification because the body's neural system does not have a single reaction to a stimulus.

If you step off a curb to cross a street, plant your foot awkwardly, and twist an ankle, there is an immediate stab of pain, which stimulates the A-Delta fibers of the peripheral nervous system, is processed via the dorsal horn in the spinal cord, and then transmits a signal to the brain, where a motor output—the response—can be formulated.

After the immediate sharp pain we feel from an injury, the pain sensation will soon begin to change, becoming more dull and throbbing. That is the C-Fibers sending a slower message down their thinner, non-myelinated "wires," which creates a delayed interpretation from the peripheral nociceptors.

The sensory nervous system's response to a harmful or potentially harmful stimulus signals that something is wrong, which in turn causes the CNS to react. An immediate physiological cascade starts, in an attempt, depending on the injury, to contain the damage. Primary and secondary mechanisms of hemostasis ensue, followed by and overlapping an inflammatory stage at the site of injury.[36]

However, there are scenarios where there is no clear stimulus and the nociceptors have not been activated.

An extreme example is phantom-limb pain, in which an amputee experiences pain that seems to originate in a limb that is no longer there.

Though we do not yet have full understanding of this phenomenon, it is currently believed that the imprint of pain on the short-term memory—the last sensation the person felt in the limb—is so acute that pain is the only sensation the brain can associate with the affected body part.[37]

There may also be an emotional component, as the events resulting in amputation may have been traumatic.

Other scenarios such as NSLBP, fibromyalgia, and chronic pain in general are examples of pain being present in the absence of nociceptive stimulation.

## IDENTIFYING A PAIN GENERATOR

The skill of differential diagnosis is a long-studied craft that separates the good clinicians from the great clinicians. It does not matter what method, school, or expert you follow, as long as you have an efficient and consistent evaluation system to identify the tissue that is the issue, assuming there is one.

Simple tissue tensioning tests are a method of determining the type of pathology present. In some cases, an athlete has injured certain tissues, but these tissues are not painful if the person is still or is passively moved.

However, when we introduce resisted manual muscle testing, we may then reveal a contractile tissue pathology. This means that if a client has an issue with a muscle, tendon, or myofascial unit, it will most likely be painful upon resisted testing.

We often evaluate non-contractile tissues, including ligaments or joint capsules, via stress testing. The therapist will place the ligament or part of the capsule under strain by placing a specified direction of force through that tissue.

If there are disrupted fibers, this testing will disturb them, creating pain or displaying laxity of the ligament or capsule if enough damage has been done.

## DIGGING DEEPER TO FIND THE PAIN GENERATOR

In general, when dealing with an athletic injury, an event started the pain cascade. Often an identifiable injury and nociceptive stimulation was the culprit of the resulting pain or dysfunction. Finding the pain generator is the key to assessment, treatment, and prognosis.

The clinician is lost when the pain generator is not properly identified. Treatment is generalized instead of focused. The patient may get stronger or more stable and may even return to the sport or job; however, it may only be at 80-percent ability, and sometimes far less.

When the pain generator is not correctly identified, the patients may not quite get over the hump, may not regain all the movement and function they need, or may not become fully pain free.

Just as we cannot start a movement pattern in a poor position and expect to perform the rest of the movement well, if we begin the rehab-to-performance process with the wrong assumption about the root of the pain, we are unlikely to end up with a fully recovered athlete.

You should not assess pain if such an assessment is not in your skill set. However, you still need to understand the diagnosis that results from an assessment performed by another professional. You need to recognize which elements to promote or avoid to help or at least not hinder the initial rehabilitative process.

## TREATING THE PAIN GENERATOR

When we start reviewing a pain generator, it is not enough to simply treat or manage those symptoms, particularly if done using prescription painkillers to make the pain level "bearable." We must also identify, evaluate, and treat the *cause* of those symptoms.

People typically relate to that in this day of functional training and examination. For example, when I was in a clinic working with a student, we had an athlete who came in with knee pain.

I asked the student to evaluate the athlete and let me know what he found. The student came back with an elaborate evaluation of the athlete's movement dysfunctions, poor hip control, poor core stability, and foot abnormalities that were all, in his opinion, contributing to the athlete's knee pain.

When asked, "What about his knee?" he asked what I meant.

"He came in for knee pain. Did you look at his knee?"

The student stared at me and finally said, "No, but his knee pain is coming from his hip, trunk, and foot dysfunction."

That may have been true, but we needed to directly address the knee. Knee pain was why he walked into our office. There is value in decreasing a patients' pain, both physically and mentally for the patient.

We sometimes forget that when trying to get to treating the cause of pain, and we skip the obvious need to treat the source of pain…simply trying to make the person feel better.

Addressing the cause of symptoms is essential for effective long-term care of

an issue, but in the short term, decreasing pain is valuable as well.

## MAKING BIOMECHANICAL COMPROMISES

When we hurt one side of the body, we often we favor the other side, but what does this mean in terms of an athlete's rehabilitation and return to a sport?

We alter our movement patterns to compensate for the presence of pain, emphasizing the non-painful side, while deemphasizing the painful one. We need to address this as part of the rehabilitation.

Recent research suggests that such a maladaptation sometimes is not temporary, lasting beyond when the pain subsides. In fact, we may need to retrain the faulty motor program and motion segment sequencing long after the successfully treating the pain generator.

According to a study by Francois Hug and five others at the School of Biomedical Science in Brisbane,[38] participants in a foot-and-ankle plantar-flexion test reduced force production in the painful leg, while increasing it in the pain-free one.[39]

This shows that if you give people the option to favor the non-painful limb in a bilateral exercise, they will do it. However, if given a unilateral task or a task with fewer degrees of freedom, there is less ability to compensate and get off the painful tissue; they will perform the task, potentially injuring already painful tissue.

We need to be strategic about when we introduce unilateral and bilateral movements into the rehab cycle. If there is tissue damage from an injury that has not been repaired, you should expect there to be a discrepancy in force production and balance during bilateral movements.

After the pain has been mitigated and the protection of tissue is no longer needed, introducing unilateral exercises in which the conditions are the same for both sides can help rewitre the motor pattern. In a successful response, the athlete stops the default favoring of the non-painful side.

## SUMMARY

It matters that we identify the tissue that is the issue. We need to know which tissue is pathologic in order to introduce our manual therapies and modalities that have the potential to improve tissue healing in the patient.

We must understand the tissue-healing properties at work so we can improve tissue healing, but also not impede healing by using activity or interventions that may be inappropriate.

If a pain generator is not identifiable, we have a different issue. Pain that is present in the absence of nociceptive stimulation has central-mechanism origins that need to be dealt with in a biopsychosocial model.

Pain is multivariate. It is subjective, cultural, social, personal, biological, and psychological. No one approach to pain management can be all-encompassing, given the vast individuality of pain perception.

The sports-medicine clinician and sports-performance specialist need to understand the complex nature of pain management and be prepared to deal with each individual accordingly.

In the next chapter, we will explore some of our options to alter pain perception.

# CHAPTER THREE
## TISSUE HEALING AND ALTERING PAIN PERCEPTION

Pain is an individualized experience based on experiences, emotion, cultural, and social influences, and it is impossible to treat pain the same way for different patients. Understanding the physiology of pain, psychology of pain, and individuality of pain will make it easier for clinicians to select appropriate pain-mediating interventions for their athletes.

In addition to understanding pain concepts, understanding the healing properties of different tissues will help the professional calculate normal timelines for healing.

Once we appreciate the normal healing processes that occur with injury, we can recognize when things are not healing as anticipated. The clinician can then select appropriate therapeutic modifiers.

## THERAPEUTIC OBJECTIVE AND THERAPEUTIC MODIFIERS

Our goal in sports medicine is simple: return the athlete as quickly as possible to the sport, work, or life activities with the least amount of risk of re-injury. In order to achieve this, Dr. Gary Delforge describes two specific things the clinician needs to do.

These descriptions are in his book *Musculoskeletal Trauma: Implications for Sports Injury Management*; the following is a summary of his suggestions.

First, we need to establish a therapeutic objective—establishing a short-term or long-term goal. Second, we choose a therapeutic modifier or intervention that will achieve the therapeutic objective.

The therapeutic objectives, taken directly from his text on page eight, include:

- *Control hemorrhage and edema*

- *Alleviation of pain and muscle spasm*

- *Enhancement of connective tissue repair mechanisms*

- *Prevention of contractures and adhesions*

- *Enhancement of the mechanical and structural properties of scar tissue*

Therapeutic modifiers are any interventions we might use in the bridging-the-gap model to accelerate, assist, or optimize the therapeutic objective. Therapeutic modifiers might include medication, modalities, manual therapy, exercise, and sometimes even psychological interventions.

When choosing a therapeutic modifier, as covered on page 10 in his text, we must consider its effects:

- *The characteristic vascular and cellular responses during a particular stage of wound healing*

- *The specific physiological or neurological response to be modified*

- *The capability of the therapeutic modifier to effect the desired response—or the indications of that intervention*

- *The potential detrimental effect of the therapeutic agent on normal, diseased, or surgically repaired tissues—or the precautions or contra-indications of that intervention*

Dr. Delforge's ideas about identifying the therapeutic objective and the appropriate therapeutic modifier have shaped the way I choose what I do with an athlete at any point in the rehab process.

Every time I choose to use ice, to mobilize or immobilize something, use a modality such as ultrasound or electrical stimulation, a dry needle, or an exercise, I must consider the therapeutic objective I hope to assist and decide if the intervention I chose has the ability to produce the desired effects.

Next, we will look at the natural physiological and neural pathways that are activated whenever there is an injury.

## CLINICAL PEARL

- Control hemorrhage and edema—

    ### CONTROL BLEEDING AND SWELLING

- Alleviation of pain and muscle spasm—

    ### STOP PAIN AND MUSCLE SPASM

- Enhancement of connective tissue repair mechanisms—

    ### CREATE A HEALING ENVIRONMENT

- Prevention of contractures and adhesions—

    ### PREVENT A LOSS OF RANGE OF MOTION

- Enhancement of the mechanical and structural properties of scar tissue—

    ### STRESS THE TISSUE ACCORDINGLY

## PHYSIOLOGICAL RESPONSE TO INJURY

Any time there is an injury, the body undergoes a process of healing. Healing can be divided into three stages.

- *Inflammation, also described as hemorrhage and hemostasis*
- *Fibroplasia*
- *Scar maturation*

These are extremely complicated and detailed processes and I encouraged you to study not only Dr. Delforge's book for a detailed explanation, but other fundamental orthopedic science references to understand the implications for specific tissues, including nerve, muscle, tendon, ligament, articular cartilage, and fibrocartilage.

When there is an injury, there is an immediate and transient vasoconstriction in the area. Phagocytes such as mast cells, macrophages, and neutrophils invade the region. This is followed by an immediate vasodilation to bring an increase in blood flow.

Inflammatory mediators are released, such as substance P, Calcium Gene Release Peptide, bradykinin, and others. Histamine creates a cellular constriction, creating gaps in the vascular wall. Fluid escapes the vessels and permeates the surrounding interstitial space. This increased fluid shuts down the lymphatic system in the area.

Compare this to too much water flowing into a clogged sink. The clogged sink cannot get water out as fast as water is coming in and the sink will begin to overflow. In the same manner, the lymphatic system cannot get the excess fluid out of the area and edema then forms.

This is initially good, as the body is containing the injury. The phagocytes and white blood cells can contain and control the pathogens that may have invaded the area. The body "walls off" the injury to prevent infection from spreading systemically.

The body proceeds to undergo processes of subacute and chronic inflammation, eventually resulting in moving into the next stage of fibroplasia.

Fibroplasia is when the body begins to form fibrous tissue to fill in the injured tissue. Fibroblasts come to the injured area and are responsible for producing collagen.

A weaker collagen called Type III is initially formed, weaker as compared with the original, uninjured Type I tissue.

The weaker collagen is smaller in size, has weaker hydrogen bonds, and lays down in a more random organization than the original uninjured tissue. However, even though not as strong, this new collagen begins to give the area the needed structural strength and stability to heal the wound.

Complete scar maturation can take years. As we are working with someone who has been injured, one of our jobs, especially early on, is to respect the forming scar tissue, and possibly assist in the process. At the least, we should be careful not to disrupt the process by loading tissues too fast and too soon.

Maturing scar tissue needs a gradual increase in tensile forces to assist in strengthening the more immature hydrogen bonds to stronger covalent bonds, improve alignment of the fiber organization and strength of the fibers to tolerate tensile loads, and help with deposition of Type I collagen.

During the scar maturation phase, we direct our interventions at improving the tolerance of load through the tissue with low loads, progressive loading, and stretching.

If this happens too fast, re-injury occurs, sending the patient back into the inflammatory phase. This begins the cycle of chronic inflammation and increased risk of re-injury.

That is a very brief description of the vascular and mechanical changes that occur with injury.

For a more detailed understanding, refer to Gary Delforge's book. He does an excellent job of describing the specific healing processes each tissue goes through after an injury. You will find it a quality resource for learning about tissue healing.

## NEUROLOGICAL RESPONSE TO INJURY

Nociceptors are the specialized sensory receptors that detect noxious (unpleasant) stimuli. These specialized sensory receptors are known as A-Delta and C-Fibers and are found throughout the body in all types of tissue, such as skin, viscera, joints, muscles.

When these receptors are stimulated via mechanical, thermal, or chemical stimuli, the electrical signal goes to the central nervous system for processing.

When tissue is injured, inflammatory mediators—bradykinin, serotonin, prostaglandins, cytokines, and H+—are released from damaged tissue and can directly stimulate these nociceptors. They can also reduce the activation threshold of nociceptors, making depolarization more probable.

From a neural perspective, A-Delta and C-Fiber nociceptors are stimulated during injury, kick starting the ascending pain pathway. A-Delta and C-Fibers, which are first-order neurons, synapse with ascending tracts, second-order neurons in the dorsal horn of the spinal cord.

Within the synapse between first-and second-order neurons, excitatory neurotransmitters are released, including glutamate and substance P, triggering the activation of a second-order neuron.

Complex interactions occur in the dorsal horn between afferent neurons, interneurons, and descending modulatory pathways as discussed below. These interactions determine activity of the secondary afferent neurons, and therefore determine what information gets to the brain for processing.

This second-order neuron travels up the lateral spinothalamic tract to the nuclei in the thalamus, where they may synapse with a third-order neuron. The lateral spinothalamic tract also has projections to the periaqueductal gray matter (PAG), hypothalamus, and limbic system.

The limbic system includes the amygdala, thalamus, hypothalamus, hippocampus, basal ganglia, and the cingulate gyrus. These structures each have a different function in memory formation and emotion. This is where long-term memories are stored and our emotions are supported.

When peripheral nociceptive stimulation occurs, the limbic system may be stimulated via both the lateral spinothalamic tract and the spinoreticular tract, and is the reason "pain has meaning" and is individual for each person.

This is responsible for the emotional aspect of pain.

## INHIBITION OF PAIN TRANSMISSION

There are mechanisms that inhibit pain transmission at both the spinal cord level, as well as descending inhibition from higher centers.

### Gate Control Theory of Pain

We discussed the Gate Control Theory of pain in the previous chapter. This theory describes a process of inhibitory pain modulation at the spinal cord level.

By activating A-Beta Fibers with tactile, non-noxious stimuli, inhibitory interneurons in the dorsal horn are activated, leading to inhibition of pain signals transmitted via C-Fibers.

This is why a non-painful stimulus, such as touching something that hurts, decreases pain.

### Descending Inhibition

The periaqueductal gray matter in the midbrain and the rostral ventromedial medulla (RVM) are two important areas of the brain involved in descending inhibitory pain modulation. Both centers contain high concentrations of opioid receptors and endogenous opioids, which helps explain why opioids are analgesic—they make us feel good.

Descending pathways project to the dorsal horn and inhibit pain transmission. These pathways release neurotransmitters like dynorphin, endomorphin, and enkephlin, which bind with the receptors in the spinal cord, thus inhibiting the stimulation of the second-order neuron at the dorsal horn.

This complex ascending and descending pain pathway, when working properly, is what internally manages pain perception internally for each person.

The body is an incredible instrument that tries to manage pain and inflammation on its own. Anything can interfere with these natural management processes to disrupt the body's ability to accomplish this. Disease, poor nutrition, poor circulation from smoking or diabetes, psychological trauma, and more can slow or delay these processes, which is where a therapeutic modifier or intervention comes into play.

Physiological and neurological responses to injury can be an entire book in and of themselves. There are so many processes simultaneously happening in our bodies when an injury occurs.

While we have hit on several of the important concepts here, it is important to note that these processes are complex. I encourage you to dive deeper into the physiological and neurological responses to injury and would like to thank Brian Hortz, PhD, AT, for his review of this section.

In this chapter, we will delve deeper into treatment options commonly used to address relief of pain following an injury. In a later section on cupping, beginning on page 60, we will expand on healing and revascularization.

## PRESCRIPTION PAIN RELIEF

Most health care professionals are well aware that prescription painkillers and the overuse of opioids are at all-time high in the United States. Most people in pain need it to go away; they want the pain to be gone fast. The problem with some of these medications is that although they do a very good job of blocking pain, they are also highly addictive, creating a massive dependency on their use.

Educating our athletes to the fact that there are other, safer alternatives to prescription pain relief is imperative in today's world of pain management.

The American College of Physicians came out with a practice guideline in April 2017, outlining their recommendations for acute, subacute, and chronic low back pain.[40] Their top recommendations based on systematic reviews of the literature through November of 2016 for acute and subacute low back

pain patients was to use superficial heat, massage, acupuncture, or spinal manipulation. If medication is needed, they recommend anti-inflammatory medication (NSAIDs) or muscle relaxers.

Chronic low back pain patients should receive exercise prescriptions, multidisciplinary rehab, mindfulness training for stress reduction, instruction in relaxation techniques, tai chi and yoga, low-level laser therapy, and spinal manipulation.

If medication is needed, NSAIDs are again recommended, followed by medications to mediate nerve pain and antidepressant medication. Opioids should only be used as a last resort and in patients where the reward outweighs the risk.

This is an absolute testament for what we have innately known for a long time: There are many options for pain relief that should come prior to highly addictive medications. These options lie in the hands of skilled professionals who understand these concepts and can apply them through manual therapy, exercise, and other modalities.

Let us explore some of the common modalities we see in sports medicine to assist in pain control.

## RETHINKING REST, ICE, COMPRESSION, ELEVATION

In 2014, Dr. Gabe Mirkin, who developed and popularized the Rest, Ice, Compression, Elevation Theory (RICE) of acute recovery, debunked certain elements of it, most notably the immediate application of ice to combat inflammation when an athlete sustains a soft-tissue injury.[41]

People then swung the pendulum in the opposite direction, advocating never to use ice because it would delay the healing process.

We will look at each of the components of RICE and critically evaluate them as they individually relate to our acute injury management.[42]

## R = Rest

We know there may be some immediate impact on movement in the post-acute injury phase. Somewhere along the way, "rest" regrettably became synonymous with "immobilization."

At times, given the complex nature of a significant injury, immobilization may be necessary. However, in general, this often does more harm than good to the soft tissue in the long run.

Immobilization negatively affects the mechanical and structural properties of a ligament, causing joint stiffening or fibrosis. Studies have shown significant decreases in load-to-failure rates post-immobilization, as well as a reduced energy-absorbing capacity and lowered tensile strength.[43]

Immobilization of muscle following an injury has been shown to atrophy healthy muscle fibers, while early mobilization has been shown to increase capillary growth to the injured muscle

tissue, improve muscle fiber regeneration, improve muscle fiber orientation, and provide a faster return of biomechanical strength.[44]

The initial thinking was that immobilizing the patient or at least the affected area would limit further damage. This is certainly the case when an AT, emergency responder, or other medical professional suspects spinal or brain trauma, or a catastrophic injury involving one or more fractures.

Yet very few sporting injuries fall into this narrow category. While we certainly need to keep our *Do no harm* mandate in mind during the acute injury response stage, completely halting the injured athlete's movement is likely to do more harm than good.

The body requires motion if its main systems are to function optimally. A lack of movement can have a similar effect, as circulation is reduced when a person is sedentary. Stopping or restricting motion might also reduce the lymphatic response needed to remove the fluid that builds up after the injury occurs.[45]

This process is dependent on the patient. Some people scar a lot, which means you will have to move them more, and do so early. Other people scar very slowly, and you might need to slow down their progress to allow scar tissue to lay down to give more stability to the tissue.

The amount of blood present in an injury will dictate the initial treatment. When we were co-teaching Orthopedic Basic Science classes at A.T. Still University,

Eric Sauers, PhD, AT, FNATA, always said, "Blood is glue."

This is a poignant statement. If an injury is severe and there is a lot of blood in the area—internally, not externally—think of blood like glue and you will realize the joint is going to need early and aggressive mobilization once the area is stabilized.

This is what makes having a good clinician on hand during the early stages of rehabilitation so vital to the overall healing process. The clinician needs to know when to be aggressive and when to back off based on tissue-healing properties and fundamental physiology.

Other than in the case of a catastrophic injury, low-load movements that do not cause further tissue damage may be more advantageous for the overall healing process than strict immobilization.

This does not mean an immediate return to competition or training, but we should try to get patients to move in ways that do not cause pain or risk further damage to the injured area.

By staying in protected ranges of motion during active recovery, the circulatory, biomechanical, lymphatic, and other systems needed to kick start the repair process will function optimally and hopefully decrease the time it takes to return to performance.[46]

## I = Ice

The neurological system plays a key role in sounding the alarm after a trauma.

Once receptor sites detect damage, they send information to the brain on a highly myelinated pathway—think of a high-speed internet connection. The brain receives the signal, decides how to react, and sends information back down the line—see the neurological processes to pain discussed on page 50.

When we apply ice to a region, we are blocking the initial alarm signals by stimulating the mechanoreceptors that carry information about touch and temperature. These signals stimulate an inhibitory neuron in the dorsal horn of the spinal cord, dampening the pain signal to the brain.

This process in known as the Gate Control Theory of Pain,[47] discussed more on page 41, and is the underlying theoretical process to the majority of our pain interventions.

The analgesic effects of ice are beneficial in decreasing pain perception.[48] Decreasing pain has great value, but there is a lack of evidence that ice helps with inflammation and edema control.

While the scientific theory of using ice to protect the surrounding tissues sounds promising, its reality may not be as valuable as we once thought.[49] Ice was thought to lower the metabolic rate in cells that were near an injury, thus helping to preserve them and ideally to decrease any secondary injury that might occur in the area due to additional cell death post injury.

However, as we reconsider the concept of this secondary trauma being a hypoxic injury, evidence is pointing to that secondary injury as possibly being due to ischemia—the lack of blood supply—versus hypoxia, which is the lack of oxygen.[50]

It has also been noted that a decrease in temperature between 5 and 15 degrees Celsius is needed to do this.[51] The lowest temperature reported to have been achieved in human tissue is 21 degrees Celsius,[52] making this concept wonderful in theory, but not very practical.

Although the application of ice may not help in the healing process, and its use to manage inflammation is questionable, it does help with pain modulation.[53] We all know firsthand and from dealing with injuries in our clients and patients that there is value in decreasing acute pain through icing.

We use ice for pain management, which can hold a significant value to our patients. Using ice to manage pain may come at a cost during the initial stages of injury; what that cost is remains unknown at this time.

## C = Compression and E = Elevation

Compression and elevation go hand in hand in an effort to control the excess fluid that accumulates from cell membrane disruption and hemorrhage after an injury.

Again, think of blood as "glue" during an injury. The more the injury bleeds internally, the more "glue" is brought to the area.

We can manage the amount of "glue" in the region via controlled motion, compression of the area, and elevation.

Combining compression and elevation decreases volume post-treatment, thereby decreasing edema. Unfortunately, these effects may disappear within five minutes of being back in a gravity-dependent position.[54]

Wearing a compression garment of some sort may reduce swelling and is worth using post injury for edema control.

Overall, we should be rethinking not only the use of RICE for acute injury, but also the reasons behind why we use these modalities. At this time, research is pointing us more toward early, progressive, and protective range of motion, the use of ice for pain management, and compression and elevation for the short- and long-term effects on swelling.

## DRY NEEDLING

Dry needling is another core component of my practice when it comes to pain management. Some consider dry needling a form of Western Medical Acupuncture. See the references to review an article by Kehua Zhou[56] to discover how acupuncture and dry needling can coexist in a medical model.

There are many styles and types of dry needling, including trigger point dry needling, intramuscular electrical stimulation, peripheral neuromodulation, superficial, and perineural.

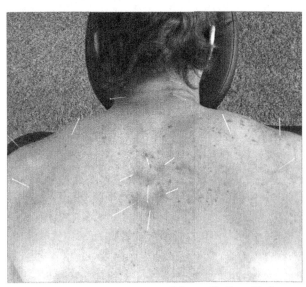

*Photo © Sue Falsone*

**Photo 3.1—Dry Needling**

*Dry needling is a skilled intervention performed by a health care professional. It uses fine filiform needles to penetrate the skin, creating a healing response in the tissue being lesioned. Tissues contributing to neuromusculoskeletal conditions can be dry needled.*

*Patients presenting with pain syndromes, movement dysfunctions, and neuromusculskeletal disorders can all benefit from dry needling.*

The first written evidence we have on the effectiveness of dry needling in Western medical journals was an article written by Karel Lewit—the same Karel Lewit who worked with Vladimir Janda and Vaclav Vojta of the Prague School, who developed Dynamic Neuromuscular Stabilization,[56] which we will cover further beginning on page 104.

Dry needling has been shown to reduce pain by stimulating the peripheral and CNS by altering the afferent information going into the system.[57]

When you break the skin with a needle and manipulate it in the soft tissues below, you create a controlled injury event.

This triggers a cascade of anti-nociceptiors and anti-inflammatory responses locally, segmentally, and systemically.[58] A-Beta fibers are also stimulated, which transmit touch sensations to the CNS, essentially dampening the pain signal to the CNS via the Gate Control Theory of Pain management.[59]

Along with the Gate Control Theory, another theory of pain control that could be at play is the Conditioned Pain Modulation.[60,61] This states that pain inhibits pain, meaning if you place a painful stimulus near something that is already painful, the second stimulus will dampen the initial pain stimulus.

These two theories of pain modulation are possible reasons that dry needling is effective in pain control.

In addition, after dry needling, the body reduces levels of stress hormones like cortisol.[62] Dry needling has also been shown to reduce the effects of myofascial pain syndrome.[63]

Dry needling can be effective far beyond providing pain relief in a specific injured area. If a person is suffering with pain and movement restriction of the elbow, for example, we could start by dry needling the tissues around the joint itself.

Then, as time allows, we might also move down the forearm toward the wrist and hand, as well as up toward the shoulder and vertebral segments around the cervical and thoracic spine.

The aim here is not just to tackle the localized pain, but also the fascial and nervous tissue that may be the source of the pain. In addition, stimulating the muscles and fascia in the motion segments above and below the injury site can improve restrictions and improve range of motion and motor control.[64]

Evidence on the use of dry needling with performance enhancement is beginning to be explored. A recent study in the *International Journal of Sports Physical Therapy* reported[65] an immediate increase in vertical jump following a session of dry needling to the gastrocnemius muscle.

Another study by Haser et al[66] found that using a dry needling intervention to healthy soccer players' quads and hamstrings resulted in improved muscle endurance, hip flexion range of motion, and significant improvement in the maximal force produced by the knee extensors.

In addition to these findings, the dry needling group had less muscle injuries during the season when compared to the control group.

Controversy surrounds the use of dry needling by health care practitioners who are not traditionally trained acupuncturists.

However, a comprehensive study by the Federation of State Boards of Physical Therapy found[67] that PTs learn four-fifths of what they need to know about dry needling while still in school. The other fifth is easily covered through additional education.

No profession should have exclusive ownership of a tool or method. Think about what would happen if EMTs were the only people who could practice CPR. Consider massage—chiropractors, osteopaths, PTs, massage therapists, and many others use massage in their practices. When we are functioning in an athlete-centered model, these controversies go away.

I have worked side by side with acupuncturists in a symbiotic, professional manner. We had mutual respect for each other and recognized that the different training we received made us unique and effective clinicians and helped us collaborate in the best interest of the patients. This, again, is how we need to function as a team with the athletes' best interests in mind.

However, dry needling is not for everyone. There are many contraindications and precautions for the use of dry needling that are beyond the scope of this text. As with any modality, if it is in the hands of an untrained or poorly trained practitioner, it can be more harmful than beneficial.

Risks are low when used by a well-trained clinician, but they certainly exist. Dry needling requires advanced training and skill for safe and effective results.

While we still have a lot to learn about how dry needling affects the body, there is already evidence to show that it causes beneficial vascular, chemical, and hormonal changes.[69]

Several studies have demonstrated that dry needling improves blood flow, prompts the development of new blood vessels, and improves glucose metabolism, all of which can accelerate rehabilitation. There is no doubt we will see more research on this tool and its application in the near future.

You will find more information on dry needling at *www.structureandfunction.net*.

## ULTRASOUND, ELECTRICAL STIMULATION, KINESIOLOGY TAPE, AND OTHER OPTIONS

### Ultrasound and Electrical Stimulation

Traditional modalities such as ultrasound and electrical stimulation have been used for a long time, are well studied and have fallen into and out of favor in the traditional physical therapy and athletic training models.

These modalities are a staple in many clinics and training rooms throughout the world. They have been shown to be effective in certain rehab and recovery situations.

The use of electrical stimulation has been shown to assist in pain management via the Gate Control Theory.[70] Many of our interventions used to manage a patient's pain are explained by this theory, developed decades ago as discussed on page 41.

The use of a conventional TENS set at a frequency of 100 Hz, a 50–100-millisecond pulse duration and a comfortable amplitude has been shown to decrease neuropathic pain symptoms in patients with CRPS when compared to sham TENS.[71] This setting has been shown multiple times in the literature and is commonly used to manage pain in clinical settings.

Ultrasound is another often-used modality for pain management.[72] Thermal ultrasound is common, using a setting that creates heat and warms the tissues, which can have a relaxing, pain-relieving effect on the patient who has muscle guarding and spasm-related pain.

Mechanical ultrasound uses pulsed sound waves to create an expansion and contraction of the gas bubbles between tissues, creating a tiny vibration and mechanotransduction into the tissue. This effect can help with pain, specifically pain caused by scar tissue or swelling.

These types of ultrasound are not to be confused with diagnostic ultrasound that creates pictures, as shown in the cupping section beginning on page 60. Diagnostic ultrasound does not have a therapeutic effect

## KINESIOLOGY TAPE

The use of kinesiology tape (KT) is en vogue, especially after the Summer 2016 Olympics, when we saw beach volleyball players wearing it in different colors and patterns. Fans of KT put it on everything for many reasons, and haters say research fails to prove it is beneficial.

The latter view is not completely true. It is very difficult to compare research

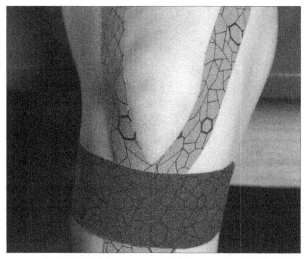 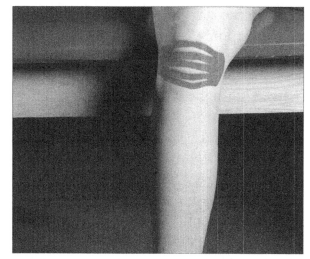

*Kinesiology tape images courtesy of TheraBand®*

**Photos 3.2a and 3.2b—Kinesiology Taping**

*While there is controversy regarding what kinesiology tape does or does not do, it has been shown consistently in the literature to decrease pain perception in the patient.*

*There is no consistent literature at this time to say the way kinesiology tape is applied makes a difference in patient outcomes, with the exception of tension. The amount of tension that has been shown in the literature to be associated with positive outcomes is 25%.*

studies on KT because the setup of each study was different. We have a lot of research on kinesiology taping; however, those studies are not easily comparable to give us a good indication for use.

If we look at KT through the lens of the various pain theories, we get differing ideas about how taping might help reduce pain. Gate Control theorists believe that by applying tape to an area, we are stimulating the hair follicles, cutaneous nerve endings, and other skin receptors, and thereby decreasing the sensation of pain.

Advocates of the circulatory theory think the convulsions in the adhesion of the tape slightly lift the skin, creating channels to promote blood flow and reduce pressure under the skin.

Finally, adherents to muscle activation theory, which states that by changing the direction of the tape—origin to insertion and insertion to origin—we can either activate or relax a muscle. These are all just theories at this stage.

The evidence is difficult to interpret, as the studies are from different sample populations, different controls, different application of tape, unclear application, and other incomparable variations.

While we are still debating many of the purported benefits of taping, there is one thing that much of the research shows the tape helping with in a statistically significant way: pain.

In 2015, Phil Page performed a mega review of recent studies and concluded that the most consistent impact of kinesiology taping is on pain reduction.[73]

The other interesting recent finding is from Craighead et al in 2015. They reported that KT increased cutaneous skin blood flow regardless of tension, and it continued for up to three days of wear.[74]

When I began teaching dry needling and cupping, I taught my first class to a group of students who were close friends and colleagues who would give me honest feedback about the course content and flow.

One attendee was Gregg Doer, who uses a lot of kinesiology taping methods, and happened to be taped during the first part of the course. When we got to the cupping section of the class, we removed the tape he was wearing and proceeded with cupping.

The next day, when reviewing at our post-cupping bruises, Gregg had a very interesting and different bruise pattern compared to those who had not been taped before cupping.

It is important to note that Gregg had the tape on *before* we cupped, not after. We could see the changed bruising pattern where the tape was before the cupping on the left side of his back in the upper two cupping spots.

In Photo 3.3, you can see the results of his cupping.

This was my first indication the taping might be something to introduce into my practice.

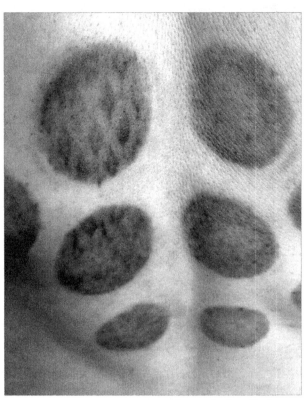

*Photo © Sue Falsone*

**Photo 3.3—Cupping after Taping**

*In this example, kinesiology tape was present on the skin prior to a cupping session. The next day when evaluating the bruising pattern, we noted the above pattern.*

*It is important to note that the kinesiology tape had been applied prior to the cupping session, not afterward. This could be explained by Craighead et al's findings that there is an increase in cutaneous blood flow for up to three days after the application of kinesiology tape.*

Tension is another interesting aspect of kinesiology taping. According to Lim and Tay (2015), the amount tension applied predicted success.[75]

Contrary to what many professionals are doing with their athletes, more tension was actually associated with smaller effect sizes.

During Page's 2015 mega review, he noted the tension level most associated with positive, significant outcomes was 25 percent. Stretching the tape as hard as you can and placing it on the skin with the maximum tension might not be the way to go according to current research.

In summary, if you are using KT on your athletes, continue the practice because it might provide pain relief and improved circulation for some people. Even if it proves ineffective for others, it certainly will not impede performance or cause pain—the worst side effect is minor localized skin irritation from the adhesive.

## USING COUNTERIRRITANTS

It is almost impossible to watch the duration of a pro sports game on TV without seeing a commercial for a hot or cold spray or a patch pitched by a big-name athlete. We place such products and others like menthol and Tiger Balm into the category of counterirritants.

The reason companies claim these work is similar to any other application of Gate Theory: When we stimulate A-Beta fibers, we stimulate an inhibitory interneuron at the spinal cord, which dampens the pain sensation to the brain. The brain literally interprets less pain from the peripheral nervous system.

Not only do A-Delta and C-Fibers transmit pain, they also send information on temperature. A-Delta fibers relay information on cold, while C-Fibers transmit the sensation of heat. If we apply a cream, patch, or spray that makes the skin feel hot or cold, we perceive this sensation instead of pain or at least a diminished sense of pain.

While it is easy to scoff at this and dismiss it as junk science, in every pro sports locker room or practice facility, you will see multiple players slathering their aching elbows, knees, or shoulders with counterirritant products.

These athletes are on multi-million dollar contracts, many of whom feel they have to play through pain. We should not dismiss their real world testing, even if the benefits are largely psychosomatic.

Indeed, there is some evidence that shows counterirritants provide at least some benefit in short-term pain management and mitigation. A Penn State study from 2016 concluded that menthol application increased blood flow.[76] Johar, in 2012, compared ice and menthol in treating delayed onset muscle soreness and concluded that menthol had a greater positive impact.[77]

As with kinesiology tape, if your athletes want to use menthol or another counterirritant as part of pain relief or management, these products may provide some benefit.

## ESSENTIAL OILS

Some of you reading this are already rolling your eyes at the idea of using essential oils for pain control. While many sports-medicine practitioners in the West are highly skeptical about alternative therapies, Eastern cultures have been using essential oils as part of a non-pharmaceutical pain management strategy for centuries.

The evidence in favor of aromatherapy is not just anecdotal. In a 2014 review, Stea et al concluded that orange and ginger oils have analgesic effects, while inhaling lavender oil reduced the amount of painkillers needed by post-operative patients.[78]

Jun et al in 2013 tested the impact of inhaling eucalyptus oil on two control groups, both of whom had recently undergone knee replacement surgery. They discovered that the patients who inhaled the oil reported significantly lower scores on the VAS pain assessment scale—a visual analog or graphic rating scale used in pain assessment. Those using the aromatherapy approach also had lower blood pressure.[79]

While it is unwise to use only aromatherapy to treat pain, incorporating the inhalation and topical application of certain essential oils might prove beneficial.

## CLINICAL PEARL

Tools for pain relief include but are not limited to:

- Controlled, protective, progressive range of motion
- Ice
- Electrical stimulation
- Dry needling
- Kinesiology tape
- Cupping
- Counter irritants
- Essential oils

## SUMMARY

Pain is a difficult thing to manage. As we have discussed, pain is conscious, subjective, and cultural.

It is personal through its link to people's memories; it is situational based on task, and there is no center in the brain to manage it. Often, pain is present even in the absence of peripheral nociceptive stimulation.

In our age of functional rehabilitation, clinicians sometimes minimize the value of managing a patient's pain.

Yet, movement will be altered in the presence of pain.[80] Therefore, managing pain should be one of our first priorities when treating a patient. This chapter identified some common and some not-so-common techniques to manage pain.

If some of the techniques are beyond your scope of practice, connect with a health care professional who can assist you when deciding if these techniques are appropriate for your client.

# CHAPTER FOUR
## MOTION SEGMENT

Once we have established the true pain generator, if we are able to isolate one, it is time to focus on the injured or dysfunctional area and help repair or restore function to it. Reestablishing this motion segment allows us to "reconnect" the injured body part with the rest of the body.

For example, we may be treating someone who has anterior knee pain. Although we are dealing with symptoms like pain, swelling, and restricted range of motion in the knee, the cause might not be originating from the anterior knee at all.

Patient symptoms may or may not have a defined pain generator. If they have a pain generator, like chondromalacia patella or patella tendonitis, it could be caused by a biomechanical dysfunction in the foot, ankle, hip, or a combination of all three. Dealing with the pain generator will address the source of symptoms, while dealing with the motion segment will address the potential causes of symptoms.

To reestablish the motion segment in preparation for more advanced movement work, we must first identify the cause of the symptoms, address them, and integrate the entire segment using corrective exercises.

The *cause* of the symptoms—the motion segment—is just as important as the *source* of the symptoms, which we will call the "pain generator."

When giving a presentation or writing an article about the importance of targeting a motion segment, I sometime get negative feedback, such as "You need to focus on the whole body" or "You cannot look at the athlete in isolation." I am not above criticism and recognize that in the course of returning an athlete to competition, we must consider health in its totality.

Nevertheless, when working to get a baseball player back on the field after surgery on his elbow and he still only has 60-percent extension in the joint, the focus must be on getting full function back in his elbow and the surrounding segments. His lumbar-pelvic relationship is important in the right context, but it is hardly the priority at that point.

One of the benefits of deploying the continuum we are exploring is that it gives a blueprint for targeting the most important factors in an athlete-centered model.

While being cognizant of the big picture and holistically looking at the mind and body, we are all professionals in the real world of caring for our clients.

There are not enough hours in a day to treat even one athlete's entire body from head to toe during every visit, let alone when working with multiple clients.

When working through the *Bridging the Gap* system with professionals who look at the care continuum the same way, I, as the rehab person, can focus my attention at the most immediate body part needing attention—in the example above, the elbow joint—while my colleagues can work on lumbopelvic hip coordination another time. The professional team deploys each person's strengths in the best interest of the athlete.

The concept of motion segments is broad. We define this as body parts and the structures between them that need focused attention before integrating with the full kinetic chain or bodywork you plan to do. It does not necessarily mean an upper or lower extremity, as a motion segment can span the entire body.

The motion segment you need to address for a particular person with a specific dysfunction might be different from the next patient with the same diagnosis.

A motion segment can be defined as a fascial line, multiple body parts in a row, an upper or lower extremity, the spine, or more.

If the pain generator section of the bridging-the-gap model looks at addressing the *source* of the symptoms, think of the motion-segment section as addressing the *cause* of the symptoms. While we address the causes of the symptoms in other parts of the continuum, this section focuses on other contributing and limiting factors to movement patterns post injury.

If you concern yourself with the total body right after injury, you might miss important details near the injury that will affect the function of that segment and, therefore, the efficiency of the whole being.

We need to spend time at the motion segment so we do not allow the body to compensate its way to the movement stage, ingraining compensatory movement patterns that may work short term, but could be problematic in the long run.

A baseball player I worked with years ago dislocated his elbow, a traumatic dislocation that needed significant surgical repair. After the surgery, we worked on swelling control, pain management, and eventually range-of-motion activities.

While his elbow mobility was coming along fine, he was not appropriately moving the affected arm in relation to the rest of his body. He kept it near his side and flexed and extended his elbow or rotated his hand only if prompted. When we asked him to reach for something in front of his body or off to the side, he was not able to do it.

It became apparent that the main problems moving forward in his rehab were not coming from his elbow, which was the pain generator. There were significant motion-segment issues because he would not let his arm leave the side of his body. His shoulder soon became the biggest concern.

In this example, his upper extremity was the motion segment, and we had a big problem on our hands. If he did not start using the entire motion segment when reaching, he was going to end up with a stiff shoulder…and that is exactly what he got.

Although this chapter will explore how issues in one part of the anatomy can have profound effects elsewhere, the real focus for us is to identify the main motion segment that is the root of your client's problem.

The motion segment must be in working order to be properly integrated into total-body activities. In the example above, there is no way the athlete would be able to use his upper extremity to swing a bat if he could not even reach for his morning coffee.

As we progress in the book, we will layer on more total-body and mind-body concepts for your evaluation.

## LOCALIZED SYMPTOMS DO NOT MEAN IT IS A LOCALIZED PROBLEM

Consider this story of a baseball player sidelined with a labrum tear in the shoulder of his pitching arm. After our conservative rehab, he was not back to full function and continued to have pain when pitching. It was clear he was headed to surgery.

One day in the training room, I saw him sitting on a table working on a toenail. He had a severely ingrown toenail on the big toe of his right foot—the same side as his throwing shoulder injury.

Bear with me for a moment while I make the connection. He had been struggling with this toe ailment for several weeks; it started before the symptomatic shoulder.

Imagine that it hurt him to push off the toe to deliver a pitch, so he had to make an adjustment to get off the painful ingrown toenail. To compensate, he unconsciously started turning his right foot outward when he pitched.

This slight external rotation of his right foot allowed some freedom at the foot and ankle, rolling though his midfoot, and taking pressure off the painful toe.

However, to achieve external rotation of his foot, he needed to externally rotate his hip. This external rotation of the hip also caused an opening of his lumbo-pelvic-hip complex.

Because of the lower-body external rotation, his arm lagged slightly behind his body, causing some unwanted horizontal abduction of his shoulder during the arm-cocking phase of throwing.

While starting from an undesirable position, he needed significant eccentric strength in the upper extremity to slow down the arm as it quickly moved from this position through the acceleration phase of throwing.

Could this excessive horizontal abduction and poor positioning in the cocking phase of throwing irritate a possibly already torn, asymptomatic labrum, making it symptomatic and thus requiring surgical intervention? Quite possibly.

There are surely many reasons this player's shoulder became symptomatic. However, this was a seemingly "insidious onset of shoulder pain," meaning that for no reason, his shoulder began to hurt.

There was no change in his pitching schedule. He was not working on a new pitch and there was no change in his training. Is it not possible that a seemingly innocuous, although irritating toe issue either caused or contributed to a more serious and debilitating shoulder injury?

This lower-extremity problem could have created a domino effect of dysfunctional compromises that eventually led to an upper-body injury as the new motor pattern became his default for pitching.

Movement assessments are a way to pick up dysfunctional compromises before they become more serious. We will discuss a few assessment options in the next section.

## MOVEMENT ASSESSMENT

Movement assessment is a broad topic. No single movement assessment has proven to be better or worse than others. Results are dependent upon a clinician's or strength coach's assessment experience, and are certainly a combination of both art and science in assessing movement.

There are many ways to assess or screen movement, some being more objective than others. The following descriptions are a sampling of assessment techniques I have used; however, this list is not exhaustive to what I use daily, or what is currently available in the field of assessments.

As you read that section, think about how you assess movement and consider if there is a way you can improve or change your movement assessment moving forward.

## THE FUNCTIONAL MOVEMENT SCREEN AND THE SELECTIVE FUNCTIONAL MOVEMENT ASSESSMENT

When trying to identify faulty motor patterns and the restrictions that can cause them, it can be difficult to know where to start. Fortunately, Gray Cook, Lee Burton, and the Functional Movement team have given us an objective test to assess movement quality. The FMS provides a way to evaluate movement with seven simple tests and minimal equipment.

The SFMA builds on this by giving formal breakouts and movement reduction for each pattern. This helps clinicians scale the fundamental movements back to their elemental parts for further discovery.

I was in the second-ever SFMA course and continue to incorporate it as well as the FMS in my practice. These screens and assessments are simple, effective, and universal, whether you are dealing with a pro athlete, weekend warrior, or untrained or detrained client.

If you need a quick, standardized, and repeatable method to highlight the motion segment that is causing a client's issue and hampering the return to competition, the FMS and SFMA are great starting points.

In addition to identifying limited patterns, they will help you uncover weaknesses, imbalances, and asymmetries that, if left unchecked and unresolved, could possibly increase injury risk and compromise athletic performance.[81]

All movement assessments come with their fair share of limitations, and the FMS and SFMA are no different.[82,83,84] However, when we can make a movement assessment objective, it gives us a way to compare our clients to themselves at different points in time.

Data collection, interpretation, and usage is something many organizations struggle with—it is a "holy grail" of metrics that could predict who gets injured and who doesn't and is the quest of every professional and college team.

However, in the absence of gross data, we can always compare an athlete to themselves. Any large change in metrics for an athlete is a red flag; whether that change is initially viewed as a positive or negative doesn't matter. A large increase in range of motion from season to season is a red flag, and a drastic change in body composition from year to year is a red flag.

Red flags may or may not end up being a problem. But they are enough of a change for me to take note and to monitor and to put the large change in perspective with everything else that is going on with the athlete.

At a minimum, assessment for movement gives us a baseline for each athlete that we can then monitor and deal with if necessary.

We will build on this discussion of the FMS and SFMA in the next chapter on psychomotor control.

## THE JANDA APPROACH

Vladimir Janda was a physician from the Czech Republic who contracted polio and had post-polio syndrome his entire life. He dedicated his work to pain syndromes and locomotion, muscle testing, and function.

He is the person who created the concepts we know as the Upper-Crossed and Lower-Crossed Syndromes used during postural assessments. You will find a longer description of these Syndromes in Appendix Four.

Janda identified six basic movement patterns he felt defined a person's overall ability to control movements.[85] These six are hip extension, hip abduction, trunk curl-up, cervical flexion, shoulder abduction, and the pushup.

He thought the order in which muscles fire to perform these movements and any compensatory patterns are clinically of value, which we will discuss more in Chapter Five, Psychomotor Control.

Janda also taught that the ability or inability to start these movements from a proper position gave the clinician information on the patient's motor control.

Janda was a proponent of breathing assessments—looking at synergistic dominance of accessory breathing muscles when a person is inhaling and exhaling.

His other assessment considerations included muscle-length testing to identify muscles prone to tightness or weakness, which set up the concepts for his Upper- and Lower-Crossed Syndromes. He also felt that a soft-tissue assessment via palpation was an important contribution to a person's movement-quality examination.

In Appendix Four, you will find a chart for documenting the Janda Assessment, including the six tests, posture, and breathing assessments. This chart is included for your convenience when implementing the Janda Assessment.

## ROLLING ASSESSMENT

Assessing developmental milestones such as rolling and crawling may or may not be valid when assessing adult orthopedic movement. Assessing movements such as rolling might give us information that could be of value when working with rotary athletes such as golfers, baseball players, or tennis players.

A rolling assessment can give the movement specialist information on the person's ability to produce coordinated movement between the upper extremities, trunk, and lower extremities.[86]

However, issues with bilateral rolling patterns are more of an indication of dynamic neuromuscular sequencing issue, rather than a true weakness. Although validity, intra- and inter-rater reliability, and injury prediction implications are not known about this assessment, it may provide useful information on multiple levels of mobility, neuromuscular control, and sequencing of rotational movement.

## POSTURE ASSESSMENT

Many people would not look at a static postural assessment as a form of a movement assessment, but I believe they fall into the same category. If your friend asks, "How do I get to the airport?," your first question would be "Where are you?" You cannot determine directions if you do not know your starting point.

This is how posture relates to movement. Static posture is where all dynamic movement originates.

Simple things like a postural grid and plumb line or higher technology devices such as X-rays or 3D analysis are all acceptable forms of postural analysis.[87]

Each method presents its own limitations, including cost, time, and even radiation exposure. Validity of each method has yet to be determined and interpreting meaningful information is often left up to the clinician.

Again, Vladimir Janda's Upper- and Lower-Crossed Syndromes may be of value to assist the professional in determining what information is meaningful from a postural assessment.[88]

## STRENGTH TESTING

Health care practitioners grade strength according to a system created by Florence Kendall (1910-2006). In her groundbreaking book, *Muscles: Testing and Function with Posture and Pain*,[89] which had five editions, Kendall outlines the importance of muscle strength and describes how to improve it based on the reason for the weakness. She gave clinicians an objective way to test and grade strength, recognizing that normal movement would be impossible if a person did not have normal strength in a muscle.

The details of muscle testing are intricate, and I direct you to her book for further understanding of these concepts. However, in general, we grade muscle strength on a scale from zero to five.

A muscle can either work against gravity or not. If a muscle cannot contract against gravitational forces, the highest grade is a two, which is poor in Kendall's muscle-strength scale.

If a person is unable to produce movement in the horizontal plane but the clinician can see a visible tendon or feel a palpable muscle contraction, the patient is given a grade of one, which is considered "trace." If no muscle contraction is felt or seen, the grade is a zero.

Strength coaches might find these grades hard to believe, but people present with these all the time when in pain or immediately post injury or surgery.

Grades of three—fair—are given if the person can fire a muscle against gravity without resistance. If the client can handle some resistance at the end range of motion of the test position, a grade of four is issued, a "good" score.

If people can hold the test position with strong pressure against what is called a "break test," this is scored a five, which is considered normal.

We address strength locally, at the site of injury, and throughout the motion segment post injury once it is safe to do so. This type of strength testing and training is fundamental to being able to perform activities of daily living and has very little to do with performance.

When people cannot move a limb against gravity, they certainly will not be able to perform any type of fundamental athletic movement. Proper strength of each individual muscle is a precursor to being total-body strong from a performance aspect. We will discuss strength performance in Chapter Nine.

The assessments for movement quality listed here are simply a sample of what are available to professionals to quantify movement. How meaningful this data is remains under study and there is currently no "correct" way to assess movement.

Your personal experience and education will play a large part in how you evaluate movement. Interpreting the findings of the data is also under study as people continue to try to define "efficient" movement. You will find more on this topic in Chapter Seven, the somatosensory chapter.

Every assessment finding needs to be tied to a meaningful functional limitation, goal for improvement, and targeted treatment intervention. If we do this, we will be able to keep our assessments organized and our interventions concise.

For this, I have included examples of an assessment grid I have used since I graduated from physical therapy school. These examples can be found in Appendix Two.

Utilizing this chart kept me true to making sure every objective finding I discovered in the evaluation process had a specific functional impact on the patient's life, with a specific goal we would try to attain and specific interventions that would be used in an attempt to achieve that goal.

Ensuring I did this with every patient kept me from performing unnecessary interventions and kept both me and my patient focused on an outcome for treatment.

## MANUAL THERAPY

Once you have identified the motion segments you need to address, manual therapy techniques at the adjacent segments may prove beneficial in the long-term rehabilitative process.

There are many treatment options, and there is no single technique that is "good," "bad," or "worse" than any other if performed by an experienced professional with the overall goal of restoring function.

From a clinician's standpoint, it is all about what resonates with your evaluative and treatment philosophies. Brian Mulligan's[90] techniques are no better than Stanley Paris's,[91] whose are no better than Ola Grimsby's.[92] These people are all remarkable manual therapists who have developed systematic ways to evaluate and treat musculoskeletal conditions.

Other practitioners may decide one school of thought resonates more with them as clinicians or is more applicable to their clients, and therefore will spend time studying that methodology. However, these are all effective when applied appropriately.

If you do not have manual therapy in your skill set, befriend a manual therapist to whom you can refer your clients as needed.

While we all need to leave our credentials at the door to focus on the patient, in this case it is helpful to look for people who have letters after their names such as COMT and FAAOMPT. These qualifications designate clinicians who have spent significant time studying a manual therapy discipline—they could be more useful to you and your clients.

Licensed massage therapists are also valuable to consult at this point in the continuum.

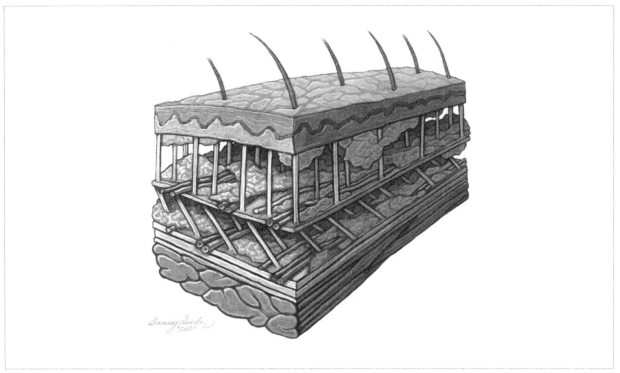

© *Danny Quirk*

**Figure 4.1—Superficial Fascia**

*Superficial fascia is made of collagen and elastin and has an irregular arrangement. It separates muscle from skin and allows normal gliding to occur between the two layers. It is innervated, which means it has the potential to be a pain generator.*

*Every cutaneous nerve has to pierce this layer to get to the skin, so stiffness of this tissue can have nerve pain implications.*

## FASCIAL AND VISCERAL MANIPULATION

When thinking about how to intervene with a motion segment, you could also consider fascial and visceral manipulation. Fascial evaluation is an up-and-coming area of study and should be a part of your future education plans.

Fascia is connective tissue that forms webbed layers over, in, and around organs, bones, muscles, and blood vessels. Rather than anchoring local structures as ligaments and tendons do, fascia runs across multiple motion segments and is integrated in various layers throughout the body.

Fascia is the true connective tissue that links us together. The following are three primary types of fascia, which are often targeted by different massage techniques and mobility tools due to their varying depth underneath the skin:

- *Superficial fascia*

- *Deep fascia*

- *Subserous fascia*

### Superficial Fascia

Directly under the skin there is a layer of superficial adipose tissue. Under that is a layer of deep adipose tissue. The tissue dividing these two layers is called the superficial fascia. This layer is made up of irregularly oriented collagen and elastin fibers. It is very elastic in youth, with diminishing elasticity as we age—hence, why we get wrinkles.

The superficial fascia supports the skin, contains blood vessels, and separates the muscles from the skin, allowing appropriate sliding between the muscles and skin during movement.[93] It is made of collagen and elastin, with enough elastin to prevent it from being a force transmitter. However, it is innervated, which means it can be a pain generator![94]

Every cutaneous and sensory nerve must pierce the deep and superficial fascial layers to get to the skin. If the superficial fascial layer becomes stiff, the nerve can become trapped and then irritated with movement.

Nerve pain can be created with movement, yet MRIs, nerve conduction velocity tests, and electromyography (EMGs) are negative because these diagnostic tests cannot recognize fascial stiffness. These patients are told they are "fine" and that all tests are negative, yet if we look to the superficial fascia, we may find the answer to a person's pain.

### Deep Fascia

The deep fascia is more dense, fibrous, and organized than superficial fascia and is in direct connection with the musculoskeletal system. The deep fascia and the deeper membranous layer of the superficial fascia are fused in some areas of the body, such as over bony prominences and over the palm and soles of the feet. That is why it is difficult to "lift" the tissue of these areas with your fingers.

The deep fascia assists in force transmission during muscular contractions and is divided into two categories: aponeurotic fascia, such as the thoracolumbar fascia, and epimysial fascia. Epimysial fascia is strongly connected with muscles such as the deep muscles of the trunk, and assists in force transmission between synergistic muscles.[95]

Recognizing deep fascia as a force transmitter will put a major wrench into the traditional way strength training is performed and movement is taught throughout the world. Deep fascia will transmit force not only in the same motor unit, but also across synergistic muscles,[96] playing a key role in defining "total body movements."

The perimysium of the muscle appears to be continuous with the tendon, contributing further to its role in force transmission.[97] Knowing that the deep fascia plays a significant role in force transmission is a huge step forward in performance-enhancement programming.

### Subserous Fascia

This third fascia type is located between the internal layer of deep fascia and the serous membranes that line the body's cavities, wrapping around organs and providing support.[98] This kind of fascia is addressed in visceral manipulation, which we will discuss in the next section.

As we continue to learn about the body and how it works as whole, the concept of individual structures is diminishing and the idea that things are anatomically connected across the body is emerging.

Using this idea of interdependent regions, all living tissues should slide and glide next to each other, with minimal or no impedance. Not only should anatomical structures function properly, they should function well in relation to the structures next to them and farther up and down the chain.

To use the earlier example of knee pain, this means if the fascia or any of the soft tissues above the knee on the anterior or posterior sides are impeded, such as in the quads and hamstrings, they will tug at the structures of the knee, potentially causing pain.

The same goes for excessive stiffness in the gastrocnemius and soleus muscles and any of the ligaments and tendons of the lower leg. This chain can go all the way down to the foot, where tight plantar fascia can be a contributor to knee pain, and up to the hip flexors and glutes.

This is also true of restrictions in the fascial layers that overlie the muscles, tendons, and ligaments in the motion segments above, below, and to the sides of the knee.

We cannot just look at localized pain or symptoms to fix our patients' issues and restore them to full capacity.

It is only by finding the roadblocks in the soft tissues and fascia throughout the system that we can take advantage of the latest applied research and not only solve a specific issue, but also improve tissue health and overall performance.

There are various ways to work on soft-tissue restrictions, adhesions, and scar tissue. No technique is right or wrong, and all techniques are appropriate given the clinician's expertise and education.

As you begin to classify your own interventions into various categories of bridging the gap from rehab to performance, you might see where a significant amount of your expertise lies.

You can then identify where you need more experience or need to create relationships with colleagues who have expertise in those areas. If manual therapy is not in your practice act, befriend someone who is an expert while you learn the inner workings of this type of intervention for the betterment of your clients.

The following is not an exhaustive list of soft-tissue interventions; it is an example of some of the techniques I use in my clinical practice.

## FASCIA

Manipulating fascia not only relates to the impact of our external forces on this specific tissues, but also to the way fascia relates to muscle: There are numerous ways to manipulate fascia; some feel better than others; and there is minimal evidence showing differences in patient and functional outcomes to determine which technique works best.

Since fascia is integrated under the skin and has a direct connection with muscle, some consider any bodywork to be fascial work.

Clinicians and performance coaches alike have jumped aboard Thomas Myers' *Anatomy Trains*. Myers was one of the first to talk about the concept of "fascial trains." Through his work, we have become more comfortable discussing and dealing with fascia in the musculoskeletal system. We will discuss these concepts more on page 80.

## Going Deep: Visceral Manipulation

Visceral manipulation is a specific form of fascial manipulation.

In order to be thorough, we need to reflect on how the organs are suspended within the torso and how the organs are attached to the structures we talk about and study regularly.

Have you heard of the ligament of Treitz? There is a band of smooth muscle that extends from the junction of the duodenum and jejunum—the small intestine—to the crus of the diaphragm.

This is the ligament of Treitz, which functions as a suspensory ligament. The right crus of the diaphragm is split by the esophagus running through it. This ligament is indirectly related to the esophagus as well.

To run through this anatomy:

- *The left and right crus of the diaphragm run down to L2 and L3, respectively, and some believe that this attaches even lower on the spine.*

- *The psoas goes up to L1—the diaphragm also attaches to the psoas.*

- *The hip flexors both attach to the lower back and diaphragm, and the diaphragm attaches to the back and the small intestine via the ligament of Treitz.*

Given these multi-point soft tissue and organ fascial connections, why are we still isolated in our thinking and solely focused on muscles? Why do we not deal with this ligament or the small intestine when looking at hip and lower-back issues? Why do we not associate digestive issues with somatic problems?

I think it is because this involves viscera, and viscera is scary for the average musculoskeletal therapist and strength coach. The above is just one example of how the viscera directly attaches to the musculoskeletal system, and if we are to thoroughly understand the musculoskeletal system, we have to be cognizant of how important fascia is in movement and its relation to viscera.

When dealing with fascia, we have no choice but to look at how this tissue interacts with the organs. In other areas of medical practice, we are more comfortable with the relationships between the organs, viscera, soft tissues, and the

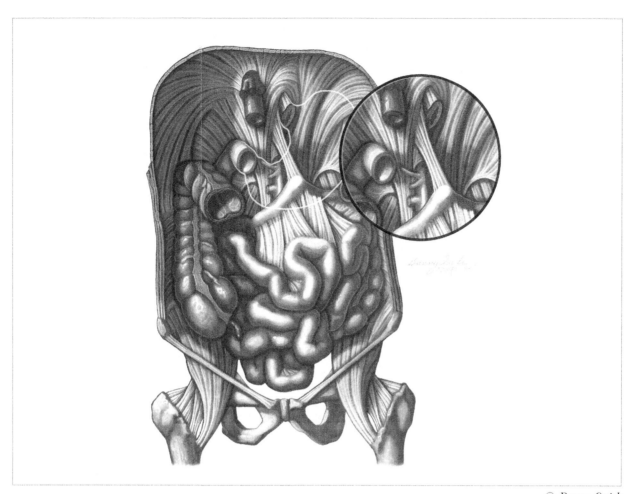

**Figure 4.2—Ligament of Treitz**

*This ligament demonstrates one example of how the organs are suspended within the body and are attached to somatic structures.*

*Knowing there is a ligament that directly connects the small intestine to the diaphragm broadens our thought process. Ten years ago, we were concerned with lumbar stability; then we realized thoracic mobility and hip mobility were an important part of this equation.*

*Soon we understood that breathing had huge implications on the thoracic spine and psoas via its anatomical connections. And now we recognize that the diaphragm has direct, ligamentous connections to organs.*

*This is just one example where we can see that organ mobility or lack thereof can have a direct effect on musculoskeletal structures, and vice versa.*

symptoms that dysfunction can produce than we typically are in sports medicine. This is particularly true of somatic pain. For example, in internal medicine, we know that stomach dysfunction or inflammatory conditions such as GERD can cause esophageal pain.

Similarly, kidney stones manifest themselves as lower-back pain. In cardiology, one of the common indicators of a heart attack is pain in the chest and the left arm. We need to apply similar holistic thinking about the relationships between various body systems and segments when we treat physical problems.

One of my most profound *aha!* moments with visceral manipulation came when I attended a course with a friend who had earlier had a surgical repair of a degenerative disc condition. Although she had progressed since the surgery, she was probably only 80 percent healed and still suffered from bouts of random, moderate pain, both in her low back and in her groin.

During one of the breakout sessions, we were to perform a sigmoid colon manipulation technique on each other. As I began working on the area our instructor highlighted, it was clear I had inadvertently stumbled on the point that was at the root of my friend's pain.

After several follow-up sessions with a visceral manipulation specialist, she regained more function and the pain stopped coming in waves—something three years of traditional therapy had not been able to achieve. This showed me firsthand how transformative it could be to target the viscera when dealing with motion-segment issues and pain.

Multiple studies demonstrate this connection.[99] Simply addressing hip mobility, nerve issues, and core stability is not always enough when dealing with a chronic lumbar spine complaint.

You do not need to know how to evaluate or treat viscera and fascia, or understand the relationships between them and other soft tissues. This is a highly specialized evaluation and intervention, so you should get to know someone who understands it.

Your referral might discover if the viscera and fascia are contributing factors in a soccer player's sports hernia or a golfer's low back pain. We need to remember to treat the source of the symptoms and the cause of those symptoms as well.

There are several pioneers active in the field of fascia research. If you have not heard of the following people or read their work, put their books on your reading list. All of these people have been highly influential, not only in the study of fascia, but also in informing us how to apply their research in clinical settings.

## The Steccos

Italian physiotherapist Luigi Stecco has been a forerunner in fascial anatomy research for decades. In recent years, his daughter, Carla, and his son, Antonio, both MDs, bolstered his work in this field. The Steccos' pioneering discoveries and recent research have shown that significant force generated by muscle contractions are not distributed to these muscles alone, but also along fascial lines.[100]

The Steccos have classified the body into different segments and each of those segments has different myofascial units. Myofascial vectors of movement come together at each segment for each myofascial unit, forming what the Steccos call "centers of coordination."[101]

From a rehab perspective, this is interesting because these centers of coordination align with myofascial trigger points and acupuncture points.[102]

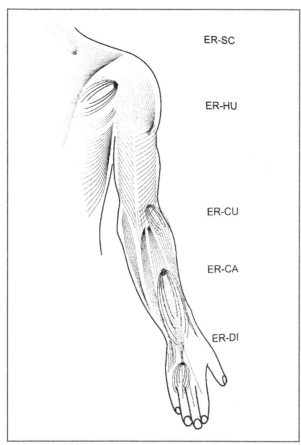

*Image from Fascial Manipulation for Musculoskeletal Pain. Used with permission.*

**Figure 4.3—The Stecco Classifications**

*The myofascial vectors of movement as defined by Luigi Stecco and family*

This reminds us how powerful these areas can be as different disciplines at different points in history have shown these areas to be important. These myofascial lines run along the entire body and demonstrate the need for a global view of fascial manipulation and treatment that does not stop at the end of a motion segment.[103]

Another key component of Stecco's work focuses on the causes of fascial stiffness. Research has shown that hyaluronan (HA) is produced by cells called fasciacytes, which are located on the inner layer of the deep fascia.[104]

Hyaluronan is present between the deep fascia and the underlying muscles, as well as throughout connective tissue surrounding a muscle and its individual fibers. This HA within the deep fascial layers allows for appropriate gliding of adjacent tissues. When this density is altered, the gliding is changed and could contribute to myofascial pain and dysfunction.[105,106]

There is a significant difference between an adhesion, densification, and scar tissue. Adhesions are created when two surfaces are not gliding appropriately in relation to each other. Densification refers to the alteration of viscosity of loose connective tissue between the deep fascial layers.

Scar tissue is an actual change in collagen make-up due to an injury. Type III collagen is laid down in an area of injury after that region goes through the inflammatory process. As discussed earlier, Type III collagen has weaker covalent bonds, smaller fibers, and random fiber orientation when compared to the original Type I collagen that was present in the soft tissue prior to injury.[107]

This leads to a conclusion that tool-assisted mobility work and massage may not be "breaking anything up," but is simply elevating the temperature of HA, thus improving the density of this lubricant, decreasing stiffness, and improving mobility following the soft-tissue techniques.[108]

While there are different theories as to why any type of instrument-assisted soft-tissue mobilization works, as covered more on page 83 later in this chapter, a simple tissue temperature increase might be what we need to decrease pain and improve function in our patients.

When we perform massage techniques or use soft-tissue mobility tools, we increase the temperature of the HA lubricant, improving its viscosity and thereby improving the gliding between the fascial layers and the muscle fibers. Better gliding decreases the subjective "stiffness" our patients feel.

Heating the fascia can decrease the viscosity of the deep fascial layers and improve the response to stretch and recoil.[109] This enhanced response could decrease hysteresis, the amount of energy lost during a loading cycle.

If we decrease the amount of energy loss in a loading cycle, we make movement more efficient. This could justify the need for a pre-activity "warm-up," simply based on tissue temperature.

The viscosity of the HA running between muscles and fascia and within deep fascia has a profound effect on the elasticity or rigidity of the tissue.

If the fluid is at its normal viscosity, it should glide over the muscles and enable them to contract to their full potential without pain.

However, if the fluid viscosity is altered, the fascia can impede muscular contraction, impacting power production, impeding movement and, in some cases, causing pain.[110]

The main implication for therapists is that when we are performing fascial manipulation, we are addressing soft-tissue adhesions that restrict mobility and also changing the viscosity of the fluid that determines the elasticity of the fascia.

## Anatomy Trains

Thomas Myers crystallized his work in the seminal book *Anatomy Trains.* Myers was influential in dispelling the myth that the body's tissues work in isolated sections. His work popularized the previously unacknowledged fact that fascia forms an interrelated, body-wide network that significantly impacts movement quality and function.

Instead of looking at bodies as compartmentalized units, Myers illustrated that we are composed of myofascial chains. He credits Ida Rolf, the creator of Rolfing, for inspiring his work with her phrase, "It is all connected through the fascia."

If the fascia are correctly sliding and gliding and have normal elasticity, myofascial forces are transmitted along the lines to their maximum potential.

However, if there is a lack of responsiveness anywhere along the fascial line, it hinders force transmission. Stiffness in one place influences the tissues up and down the line.

The Kinesis Myofascial Integration Model—a movement education and manual therapy protocol with 12 progressive deep bodywork sessions—is the practical manifestation of Myers's lines and structural integration theories.[111]

Krause et al[112] performed a systematic review of the literature, looking for evidence of these myofascial chains based on force transmission.

While there was moderate evidence to show force transmission at three transition areas in the superficial back line, front functional line, and the back functional line, evidence was difficult to compare due to different methods of force transmission and outcome measurements.

We need further studies in vivo to identify the anatomical validity versus theoretical models of force transmission in these "anatomy trains."

## Fascial Fitness

Robert Schleip is the director of the Fascia Research Project at Ulm University in Germany and is the Research Director of the European Rolfing Association. Schleip is another major contributor to the fascial anatomy field, specifically regarding how the mobility, contractility, elasticity, and hydration of fascial layers affect human movement and sports performance.

In addition to looking at the physiology of fascia, Schleip and his fellow researchers are exploring the relationship between its physical qualities and the nervous system. They have found a close connection between the autonomic nervous system and fascia, which means stimulating sensory receptors can impact tissue tone.

When treating our athletes, we need to be mindful of that tie between the neural subsystems and the tissues we are attempting to restore to full function.[113] Furthermore, multiple researchers agree there is a big presence of sensory nerves in fascia,[114,115] making it a vital sensory organ for stretch, sheer, and strain, as well as proprioceptive communication.

Another takeaway from Schleip's work is his Fascial Fitness collaboration with Divo Müller, Thomas Myers, and the Kinesis group. This work applies the latest fascial research to a more thoughtful and holistic approach to training, which focus on more than muscle stimulus and response.

According to the Fascial Fitness approach, fascia is described in terms of its ability to store and release energy, making it a vital, active component in the mobility and stability of the entire musculoskeletal system. Considering that the tissues surrounding a muscle and its individual fibers are made of epimysium, endomysium, and perimysium fascia, it makes sense that the deep fascial layers contribute to force transmission.[116]

If a training load is appropriate and recovery is sufficient, fascia responds in a way similar to the muscles, tendons, and ligaments, becoming stronger, more elastic, and more powerful.

However, if the load is too great, recovery is inadequate, and variability is too low, fascia becomes restricted, adhered, and less elastic. This means it can no longer transfer the forces generated by the muscles, reducing the impact of improved muscle strength.

To empower coaches, therapists, and the athletes they work with, Fascial Fitness provides guidance on fascial hydration, plasticity, coordination, and resiliency. It also shows specific exercises designed to improve the function of the fascial layers within virtually any type of movement pattern.[117]

## BALANCING THE THORACIC SPINE, GUT, AND AUTONOMIC NERVOUS SYSTEM

The connection between certain areas of the body and neural subsystems is another consideration when addressing dysfunction in a particular motion segment. For example, the thoracic spine and gut are intrinsically linked to the balance of the autonomic nervous system.

In earlier days, I prescribed fairly aggressive thoracic spine mobilizations to any client who showed diminished thoracic rotation or extension.

As I learned more about the connection between this area and autonomic nervous function, I discovered that over-stimulating or over-mobilizing the thoracic spine can potentially exacerbate issues by stimulating the systemic fight-or-flight response. In such cases, those efforts may have been helping with thoracic mobility, but at a cost of over-stimulating the sympathetic nervous system.

It is better to have clients perform more subtle spine exercises that focus on diaphragmatic breathing as they ease into rotation. This will alleviate stiffness that may be compromising spinal and shoulder mechanics without repeatedly pushing the "go" button on the sympathetic nervous system.

Breath-centric thoracic spine work also allows us to remove restrictions in other parts of the system, such as in the ribcage, neck, serratus anterior, posterior, and lats. The controlled breathing encourages the parasympathetic "rest and recover" response that can help release tension caused by pain.

The gut is another area closely linked to the sympathetic and parasympathetic seesaw. Jill Miller from Yoga Tune Up has done a great job getting the word out about abdominal massage and how it stimulates the vagus nerve that is so important in parasympathetic response.

The vagus nerve is the longest cranial nerve in the body, running from the brain to the gut.[118] It has both visceral and somatic nerve fibers, meaning it affects both muscles and organs.

Jill's "gut smashing" techniques help liberate stiff muscles and densifications in fascia, as well as having a positive visceral and parasympathetic impact.

Since the psoas attaches in this area, abdominal massage can provide some unexpected and welcome relief to those suffering from back pain. It may even help remove blockages in lymphatic vessels that can compromise immune system function.[119]

## INSTRUMENT-ASSISTED SOFT-TISSUE MOBILIZATION

Instrument-assisted soft-tissue mobilization (IASTM) is another increasingly popular manual therapy concept we can apply to a troublesome motion segment. Though it has its origins in Chinese gua sha, modern IASTM in the United States was popularized by Dave Graston.

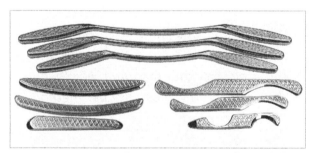

*Image courtesy of HawkGrip*

**Photo 4.1—HawkGrips Tools**

*Instrument-assisted soft-tissue mobilization (IASTM) is an advanced form of myofascial mobilization, similar to deep-tissue massage.*

*This technique enables the clinician to identify adhesions and fascial restrictions in soft tissue based on the vibrations created when a specially designed instrument is manually glided across a patient's skin.*

*Optimal function can then be restored by applying specific treatment strokes with the instrument.*

The IASTM technique uses a hard-edged instrument made of metal, plastic, or ceramic to create a shearing stress in soft tissue that advances a healing response. There is a small contact surface where emollient is used for a smooth glide, making IASTM usually comfortable for the athlete. If there is any fibrosis where the tool glides over the motion segment, it gives the clinician a heads-up that there is a tissue irregularity that needs to be addressed.[120]

There are multiple ways IASTM techniques provide mobility benefits, both in range of motion and motor control. From a physiological standpoint, the micro-trauma caused by using mobility tools recreates the body's initial inflammatory response by stimulating fibroblasts—cells that make collagen, elastic fibers, and other structures involved in soft-tissue repair.[121]

Via the theory of mechanotransduction, IASTM prompts conversion of Type III to Type I collagen, which can improve muscle and fascial elasticity.[122] One study found that tool-assisted mobility techniques also accelerated the healing of damaged knee ligaments.[123]

Mechanically, tool-assisted work removes restrictions and adhesions by creating realignment of repaired collagen tissue.[124] Fascially, the heat will impact the viscosity of HA.

There are also thought to be circulatory and vascular benefits, including reduction in edema and increased vasodilation, which allows blood to flow more easily to the affected motion segment, not only carrying nutrients, but ridding the injured area of toxins as well.[125] IASTM can also remove metabolites and hydrate soft tissues.[126]

In addition to all these positive physical effects, IASTM is thought to have multiple neurological benefits. Stimulating myofascial fibers seems to reduce tone in overly tight muscles, while also improving the mechano-transduction in the peripheral nervous system, which contributes to proprioception and sensing pain.[127]

Mobilizing with tools might also cause hyper-stimulation of the neural system, prompting a return to normal function.[128] IASTM has been a significant part of my practice since Don Chu, PhD, PT, AT, introduced me to concept in 2004. Since then, I have successfully incorporated the technique, specifically with chronic and recurrent tendon and muscle injuries.

## CUPPING TECHNIQUES AND BENEFITS

If you see the aftereffects of cupping without any explanation, you might think the patient had undergone some kind of inappropriate massage technique gone wrong. The bruising and skin discoloration is dramatic, but despite the sunset-like vivid coloration of the skin that can scare off medical and lay people alike, the benefits of this Eastern medicine practice can be remarkable.

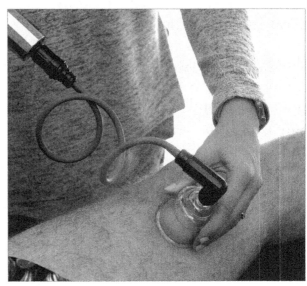

*Photo © Sue Falsone*

**Photo 4.2—Types of Cups and Cupping Machine**

*There are many types of cups and cupping machines. Ultimately, they all function the same way: utilization of negative pressure to lift tissue under the cup in an effort to decompress the area.*

*While alcohol and flame has been shown to create the most pressure inside the cup, the mechanical pump has been shown to be the most reliable method of cupping. Machines are also used in an effort to standardize pressure between treatments.*

Almost every soft-tissue treatment method relies on compression to alter how Type I and Type III collagen lays down during the repair process. Manual therapy techniques use compression to restore visceral motility and mobility and increase the viscosity of lubricating fluids in joints and in HA located in the deep fascia.

Cupping is different. Unlike compression-based approaches, cupping actually lifts skin and soft tissues into plastic or glass cups using negative pressure—at least at the center of the cup; compression does occur under the rim. It is a *distractive force* under the center of the cup, rather than a compressive one.

Cupping can be performed by using glass cups, lining the cup with alcohol, and setting a cotton ball on fire to create heat under the cup, creating negative pressure. It can also use plastic cups, with a manual pump or a twist top, both of which create negative pressure under the cup.

Huber et al[129] found that using a glass cup with alcohol produced the most negative pressure under the cup, while the mechanical pump was the most reliable. They also found that inter-rater reliability was good. It took people about 20 repetitions to go from a novice cupper to an expert cupper, meaning the skills for the technique are easy to learn.

While the mechanical effects of cupping are self-evident—people feel better after it is performed—it is still unclear why it works. However, its benefits are tangible in the alleviation of myofascial pain, improvement of circulation to injury sites recurrently or chronically injured, and enhanced soft-tissue mobility.

Practitioners of Traditional Chinese Medicine, in which cupping has been included in the art for more than 2,000 years, believe that it works by unblocking Qi and enabling this life-force energy to flow unhindered through the body.[130]

Though there is little definitive Western research on cupping, there have been multiple studies suggesting how cupping might work.[131,132,133,134,135,136]

There are two theories: a biomechanical theory and a circulatory theory.

A biomechanical modeling study by Tham showed that tension of the tissues would be highest at the center of the cup and would extend 0.4 times that of the diameter of the cup.[137] Under the rim of the cup is where compression actually occurs. This information needs to be replicated in human tissue.

The compression-to-tension change in the tissue needs to be studied to see if there is enough force at this interface to cause adhesions or scar tissue to be disrupted and remodel the scar.

More information is needed to validate not only the distraction that occurs at the center of the cup, but also the transition zone from compression to distraction, as well as how these compare to the straight compression of our manual therapy and IASTM techniques.

Very early–stage musculoskeletal elastography use has shown a decrease in stiffness in tissues during and after cupping, as well as a decompression of tissues during and after cupping in the quadriceps muscle.

Musculoskeletal elastography uses a musculoskeletal ultrasound unit to detect the amount of stiffness in a tissue. In Photo 4.3 on the following page, you can see the change in stiffness during a cupping treatment compared to before the treatment.

How long this change in stiffness lasts or how it is clinically significant remains to be seen. Detecting how stiff a tissue is can give us information about the general health of the soft tissue. In the future, elastography will give us significant information about soft-tissue interventions.

## Healing and Revascularization

Microcirculation problems have been shown to be the cause of many chronic disease processes.[138,139]

"Microcirculation" refers to the circulation that occurs between the arteriole, the capillaries, and the venules—the smallest blood vessels in the body.

When microcirculation gets disrupted due to scar tissue formation, the tissue may not receive adequate blood flow to assist in healing and nutrient transfer. The microlymphatic vessels are compromised as well, leaving interstitial fluid in the area that can cause secondary injury to the surrounding tissues.[140]

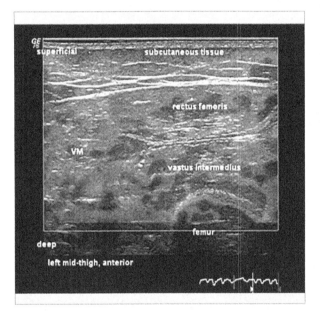 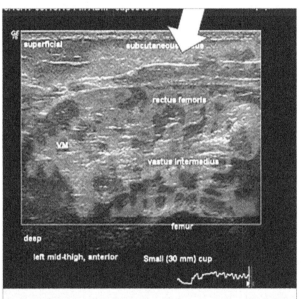

*Images courtesy of Chandi Pedapati and Dr. Inder Makin—A. T. Still University*

**Photos 4.3a and 4.3b—Musculoskeletal Elastography**

*Musculoskeletal elastography utilizes a musculoskeletal ultrasound technique to detect the amount of stiffness in human tissue.*

*Here is an example of a musculoskeletal elastography image showing the difference before and during a cupping treatment.*

*In the second picture, you can see more areas of darkness in the subcutaneous area, indicating a decrease in stiffness of the tissue.*

Muscle heals through a combination of regeneration and repair. Regeneration of the myofibers occurs by the differentiation of satellite cells into myoblasts, which form myotubes that fuse with the injured myofiber.

Scar tissue is also formed via the repair process after the initial injury. These two processes must be balanced for proper healing of muscle tissue.[141]

Revascularization of this tissue is critical after injury and occurs by angiogenesis—the process of making new blood vessels. If revascularization is inadequate, healing will be affected and can result in chronic, recurrent muscle strain.[142]

When we cup an area, blood collects in the tissue pulled into the area under the cup. Healthy tissue with a properly working microvascular system will simply dissipate this blood once we remove the external stimulus of the negative pressure of the cup. If proper microvascularization is not present, the blood stays there, and we see bruising.

In theory, the body then responds by creating new arterioles, venules, and capillaries to move the pooled blood away via angiogenesis. How long this process takes will dictate how long it takes to dissipate the bruise.

At the same time, in a process known as autolysis, the body also breaks down any damaged or unused vessels that have been contributing to limited blood flow in the damaged muscle.

The therapy can also dilute inflammatory markers by bringing more blood to the site of the cupping. In addition, a South Korean study on hypertension patients found cupping to be more effective than drugs in improving vascular filling.[143]

In the absence of research and scientific evidence, sometimes we have to turn to scientific principles to guide our interventions. While the theory of angiogenesis and its relation to cupping is uncertain, it is certainly scientifically sound.

## Cupping and Pain Relief

In thinking about pain theory, cupping may help decrease pain via the Gate Control Theory. A recent study by Walker et al discusses the discovery of a touch-sensitive nerve fiber called the "C-tactile afferent" nerve fiber.[144]

This C-tactile afferent nerve fiber is stimulated by low-velocity, low-force touch and actually inhibits pain, as opposed to the long-known C pain fiber. Stimulation of this nerve fiber may also stimulate the production of oxytocin, a "feel good" hormone. This will be an interesting area of future research regarding the use of cupping, as well as all manual therapies and pain modulation.

Cupping may positively influence several microsystems. First, it stimulates the peripheral nervous system.

Sometimes after a traumatic injury that involves a high level of pain, the sensory receptors can go haywire. The stimulation that cupping causes might act as a reset button that recalibrates pain receptors and thereby reduces lingering pain sensations.[145]

It can also reduce pain by stimulating the CNS. The excessive blood flow brought about by cupping therapy, called hyperemia, is thought to trigger the brain's release of pain-blocking neurotransmitters.[146]

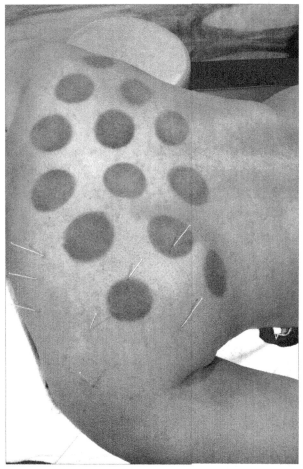

*Photo © Sue Falsone*

**Photo 4.4—Hyperemia from Cupping**

*Cupping can cause anything from slight pink changes to the tissue to obvious bruising. Pink discoloration is usually from histamine that gets released in an area any time you irritate the skin.*

*Bruising occurs when blood is brought to the area of injury via the cup; the body does not have an internal mechanism by which to dissipate this blood. Therefore, the blood sits in the area and bruising is observed.*

## Recovery Timeline

Typically, it takes between three and 10 days for the bruising caused by cupping to dissipate. Theoretically, the length of time depends on the patient's overall physiological health, which determines self-healing ability.

In fact, we can use the recovery timeline as a prognostic measure of an athlete's wellbeing. When the cupping bruising subsides in three days, it tells us that perhaps the overall systems are working well and the person's general health is good.

However, if it takes more than 10 days to dissipate, this may indicate the overall recovery might take longer. If this is the case, we could ask about volume of movement, nutrition, sleep, hydration, and smoking habits, all of which can affect the ability to heal.

A body may also be unable to bring blood to an area when we apply an external stimulus. In Photo 4.5 on the next page, you can see redness in three of the cups, but one cupped area is white.

The theory is that circulation is so poor in this area that even with external stimulation, the body still cannot bring blood flow to the space under the cup. This may be a worse scenario than bruising. In this case, the white area under the cup correlated with the athlete's pain.

Of course, before you perform any of the techniques described, you should seek proper training to use these progressions. Do not work out of the scope of your professional practice.

- *Static cup–static body*

- *Dynamic cup–static body*

- *Static cup–dynamic body*

### *Static Cup–Static Body*

This first variation is the go-to when we have concerns about a client's physiological state. We want to stimulate the process of angiogenesis in a tissue that may have compromised microvascularization.

With the static–static technique, have the athlete lie down and get into the rhythm of slow diaphragmatic breaths with a controlled inhale and exhale.

Then, place one or more cups on the affected area and leave it or them in place for about five minutes, while monitoring the skin under the cups for color change or any negative effects, such as bleeding or exudate coming through the skin. If there is any sign of this, immediately remove the cups.

In the lab, we have begun some pilot studies to begin looking at what cupping does to the soft tissue as well as the microcirculatory system. Photos 4.6a–4.6b on the following page are of a thin 25-year-old woman whose body composition measurements and weight were not taken.

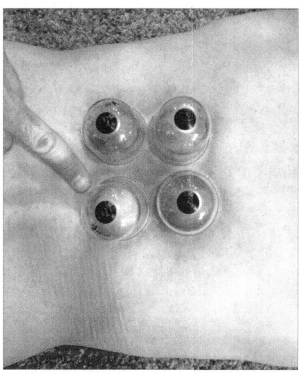

*Photo © Sue Falsone*

**Photo 4.5—Poor Circulation Shown after Cupping**

*When circulation is extremely compromised, we may see areas of white under the cup instead of red, as in the above picture.*

*Despite utilizing negative pressure, the area under the cup on the bottom left is not bringing blood to the area. In theory, this indicates a severely compromised microcirculation system and can indicate poor healing in the area due to poor capillary refill and blood supply.*

## Cupping Techniques

I use three main cupping progressions, depending on the athlete's needs and limitations, the person's experience with cupping, and the nature of the injury or condition.

In this example of a static–static technique, we see a decompression of the tissue by using a 30-millimeter cup, down to a depth of four centimeters.

We need further studies to determine what the optimal cup depth is per body part, how body composition affects the decompression, differences in gender, and other factors.

## Dynamic Cup–Static Body

If we have concerns about the fascia or other soft tissues in a particular motion segment, we might go with dynamic–static cupping. We know from the work of fascia experts that restrictions are not always rooted in a particular muscle, but can be caused or exacerbated by an adhesion anywhere along the fascia.[147]

By moving the cups, we can target different points along these lines, with the idea of not only making a positive impact on localized circulation, but also to release tension in the fascia and possibly improving fascial elasticity by increasing fluid viscosity.[148]

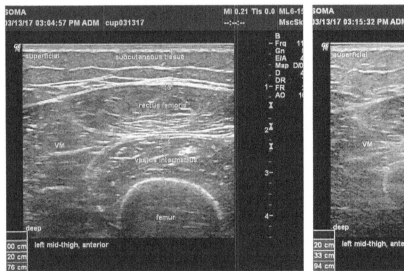 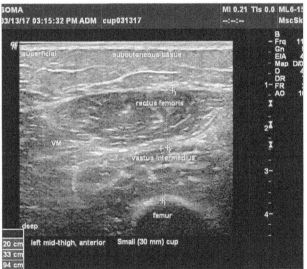

*Images courtesy of Chandi Pedapati and Dr. Inder Makin—A. T. Still University*

**Photo 4.6a and 4.6b—Musculoskeletal Ultrasound**

*The picture above is a musculoskeletal ultrasound (MSK US) image of a static-static technique being performed on the thigh of a young woman. The MSK US picture shows the distance between the layers of the muscle and subcutaneous tissue before and during treatment using a 30-millimeter cup.*

*You can see in the picture on the right that there is a 0.2 mm increase in tissue measurement at the deepest layer (vastus intermedius), a 0.13-millimeter increase at the middle layer (rectus femoris), and a 0.18-millimeter change in the subcutaneous layer.*

*Further research is needed to determine if these changes are significant, what they mean clinically, and how long these changes in the tissue last.*

In the dynamic cup–static body technique, layer the target area with lotion or cream to allow cup movement without irritating the skin. Next, place a cup, leave it a few seconds, and then move it along the fascia. This takes place while the person is stationary.

This technique is significant in my practice, as it is a way for me to periodize my soft tissue work.

We know the body generally likes periodization—we have in-season and off-season training, upper body and lower body days, pushing or pulling training sessions. We train differently and eat differently every day because the body will adapt to a changing stimulus.

If you performed the same workout and ate the same food every single day, you would eventually stop seeing body composition changes and likely experience a potential decline in performance. Yet, we perform the same type of soft tissue techniques day in and day out.

Foam rolling, massage sticks, soft tissue techniques, and IASTM are all forms of compressive tissue interventions. If for no other reason than this you decide to introduce cupping into your practice as a way to periodize your soft tissue work, that is a good reason.

In the person on whom we performed the ultrasound images in Photos 4.3a and 4.3b, we saw a decrease in tissue stiffness in the elastography during dynamic–static cupping.

Elastography uses musculoskeletal ultrasound in a way that gives us information about the soft-tissue quality by mechanically deforming tissues.[149]

### Static Cup–Dynamic Body

This type of cupping involves placing one or more cups on an area and then having the client perform a movement or transition between movements.

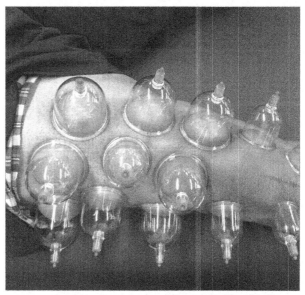

*Photo © Sue Falsone*

**Photo 4.7a—Static Cup–Static Body**

*The static–static cupping technique is used when there is a concern about the physiology of a person. You want to bring blood to the area to stimulate angiogenesis and to promote healing.*

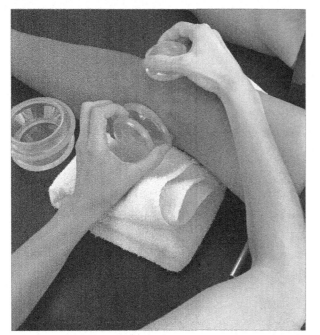

*Photo © Sue Falsone*

**Photo 4.7b—Dynamic Cup–Static Body**

*The dynamic-static cupping technique is used as a way to periodize soft tissue work. By having a technique that can decompress the tissue, you can alternate its use with compressive soft tissue techniques.*

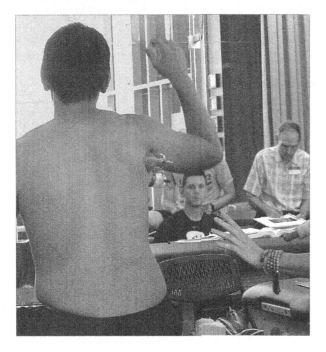

*Photo © Sue Falsone*

**Photo 4.7c—Static Cup–Dynamic Body**

*This is a demonstration of static–dynamic cupping. In this technique, cups are placed in an area and the patient moves either on alone or with assistance from the practitioner. This technique is used when there are range-of-motion limitations in an area.*

We would typically use static cup—dynamic body technique when concerned about a loss of range of motion to try to restore normal function. For example, if you are helping an athlete rehab a lower-back injury, you might place a couple of cups in the affected area and then have the person get into quadruped pose.

Once the athlete has taken a number of controlled diaphragmatic breaths, you would have the person transition into a yoga child's pose, repeating the cycle several times.

You might then add new poses or exercises or reposition the cups in a slightly different location, or use a combination of changes.

## SUMMARY

There are many ways to define, assess, and treat a motion segment. How you choose to define that segment may vary from client to client. When dealing with an injury, we need address the source of the pain and the cause of the pain.

The cause of the pain is often nowhere near the symptom of which the client is complaining. A skilled clinician needs to identify the potential influencers of pain and determine the best way to deal with them.

If this is a skill set outside of your scope of practice, befriend a clinician who can help get your athletes on the path to feeling better.

## CLINICAL PEARL

### How We Use Cupping

**Static (cup)—Static (cup)**

Used when there is a concern about the physiological ability for the tissue to heal

**Dynamic (cup)—Static (body)**

Used when periodization of soft tissue work is desired

**Static (cup)—Dynamic (body)**

Used when a range of motion deficit is present

# CHAPTER FIVE
## PSYCHOMOTOR CONTROL

Skeletal muscle makes up a significant portion of the body. These muscles can be strong, but if not firing at the right time and in the right order, strength is irrelevant—strength does not matter if it is not being applied properly.

You can have really strong glutes, but if you cannot extend your hips, you will move through your back and hamstrings when you begin running. Just because something is biomechanically strong does not mean it is neurologically preferred by the body. This is where *motor control* comes into play.

As motion segments work together to produce a movement, each muscle has a designated job if the motion is to be efficient and sustainable. Prime movers must remain prime movers; synergists must remain synergists, and stabilizers must remain stabilizers.

When a stabilizer becomes a synergist—such as with lumbar musculature assisting in hip extension, or a synergist such as the hamstrings becomes a prime mover, or a prime mover like the glutes decreases its activity because something else is doing the job—pain is often the response. This not only has long-term movement implications, but can also create abnormal joint forces that can cause harm over time.

Neuromuscular control is the fine-tuning that ensures proper posture and movement. The body is a great compensator and will adapt its function and positioning as needed.

If you need to run down the field as fast as possible because if you do not, someone is going to tackle you, your body will figure out how to get the job done. It will help you to run as fast as you can using everything it can recruit to prevent you from being tackled.

Often, the body gets away with these compensations. You may be able to use a faulty movement pattern once before injury occurs, or perhaps thousands of times. Each one of us and every compensation is different.

However, despite individualized tolerances to poor biomechanics, there will eventually be a reckoning. Over time, compensation will lead to altered movement, decreased performance, pain, asymmetries in flexibility and strength, and will further exacerbate an issue.

Think of the game Jenga, with its neatly stacked blocks. One by one, people remove a block, and the tidy stack begins to wobble and twist. Sometimes, a player makes a risky move; the stack falls and the game ends quickly.

Other times, the play goes around and around the circle, the stack twisting into a shape that makes you wonder how it is still standing. Eventually, someone takes out a block and the whole thing tumbles.

Whether a game of Jenga lasts for seconds or minutes, the end of the game is always the same: The stack of blocks falls over. Our bodies are the same.

Some athletes cannot make it one season into a professional career without injury, while others play for many years, continuing to move with poor body mechanics and yet somehow defying the odds of injury.

Eventually, no matter how resilient an athlete's body is, it will break down and injury will result from faulty positioning or movement, even if it is later in a career or life.

Our job is to help people move well so things do not get to this point. If we notice flawed patterning, we need to provide alternatives that not only correct biomechanics in the short term, but also improve long-term durability.

We need to give a body time to adapt to any changes we suggest. If you are working with an in-season athlete, it may not be the right time to try to change body mechanics. When people have developed a compensatory movement pattern, they are efficient using that pattern.

When we take the compensatory pattern away, we destabilize the system and create more inefficiency. When dealing with psychomotor issues, we need to allow the body time to adapt. This means hundreds or maybe thousands of repetitions to ingrain a new motor pattern. It is important to consider timing in your assessment and treatment.

The saying "you cannot teach an old dog new tricks" is not entirely accurate, but it is close. Learning a new skill is a conscious activity.

Everything we do to learn the new skill is focused. Every time we perform the new skill, the motor pattern becomes ingrained, creating synapses between neurons that make the pattern more automatic. That pattern eventually becomes automatic and then little conscious thought is necessary.

However, when learning a new way to do an old skill, the nervous system first needs break down old neural pathways as it is trying to build new ones. This takes more time and more repetition.

Motor control issues in athletes are best left to the off-season when the nervous system has time to adapt. Attempting to alter motor programming during a competitive season in an attempt to make the body more efficient and reduce the potential for later injury can actually have the opposite effect.

Yet if our clients are hurt, we must intervene to help them restore range of motion and motor control. At the same time, pay attention to a default to compensatory motor patterns that can make an issue worse and potentially lead to future problems.

Pain changes the plan.

## MUSCLES ARE NEVER "OFF" OR "ON"

We commonly hear practitioners say some variation of "Your glutes are not firing," or "We need to shut off your upper trap." These ideas imply that muscles can be "on" or "off" at any given time.

This is incorrect—muscles are never on or off. Actually, if we had to pick one choice, it would be that they are always on, ready to fire in case the immediate need for movement arises. This is known as the "resting tone" of a muscle.

Phrases like those are fine from a patient education standpoint. We have to make things simple so people can understand what we are saying, just as the mechanic has to make things simple for me when I take my car to the shop. I have no idea what parts of a car go where or the technical terms involved in a repair. He needs to make things straightforward for me, even though the issue is much more complicated than the sentences he may use.

The same goes for the human body and our patient education. We need to make things insanely simple so our clients have

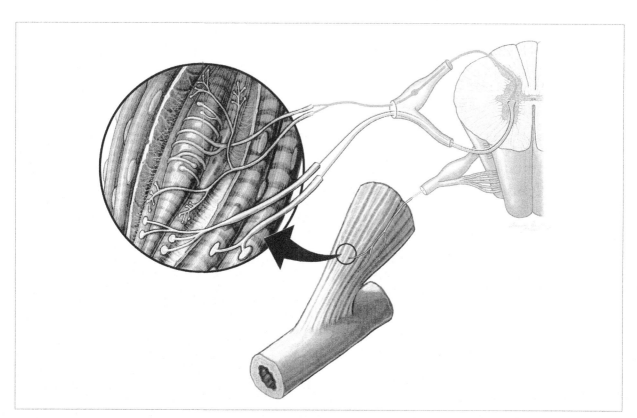

© *Danny Quirk*

**Figure 5.1—Muscle Fibers**

*Within the muscle spindle, we have intrafusal muscle fibers, which detect changes in length of the muscle, and extrafusal fibers, which contact, to maintain proper tension within the muscle as a whole.*

*This "pre-tension" keeps the body ready for movement at any given instant.*

some understanding of what is going on and how we plan to deal with the issue.

A problem comes into play when we habitually use sentences like this as professional talk among our peers. Our patient education has become our professional dialog. In doing this, things get lost in translation.

We begin to simplify the process in our minds and begin to believe that a muscle is, in fact, "off." We need to get back to the facts and use science-based conversations if we have any hope of continuing to elevate the professions and having inter-professional dialog.

## WHAT IS ACTUALLY HAPPENING?

What is happening if a muscle is firing too much or not enough?

Let us look at an example. You have certainly encountered the scenario where a client complains of tension in the upper trap or a pain in the neck region. You look at the person, maybe palpate the muscle, and then say, "Your upper trap is really firing. We need to decrease the firing in your upper trap and fire your lower trap more."

You then proceed to massage, use a massage stick, maybe ultrasound, or do other interventions to "turn off the upper trap," and do then exercises to "turn on the lower trap."

First, neurologically, we know the trapezius is innervated by cranial nerve XI—the spinal accessory nerve. All parts of the trap have the same innervation,

therefore it is neurologically impossible to fire one portion of the trap without firing the whole muscle.

However, take a biomechanical look at this. Go back to muscle anatomy 101 and look inside the muscle fiber, as seen in Figure 5.1 on the previous page.

We have an intrafusal muscle fiber that lies within the muscle spindle. The intrafusal muscle fiber detects length changes in the muscle. When stretched, it sends signals from the intrafusal fiber to the spinal cord via sensory nerves.

The spinal cord then sends a signal to the gamma motor neuron and the alpha motor neuron. The gamma motor neuron innervates the ends of the intrafusal fiber, telling them to contract. The alpha motor neuron contracts the actual muscle spindle—the extrafusal fibers, also known as actin and myosin.

If the sensory nerve of the intrafusal fiber is constantly telling the spinal cord to activate the alpha and gamma motor neurons, the "tone" of the muscle will be high from constant firing.

Then, because the body undergoes a constant balance of collagen turnover—the synthesis and lysis of collagen—the new collagen begins to lay down according to the forces placed on the tissue.

If this happens in a lengthened state due to a poor posture that may have started the whole cascade to begin with, we now have an excess of collage deposition in the lengthened state, stiffening the muscle tissue.

The upper fibers of the trapezius become chronically tonic from the sensory input of the intrafusal muscle fibers, and the tissue gets stiff due to collagen turnover.

We have a sensory issue we need to deal with by changing the posture and decreasing the sensory input to the spinal cord. We also need to work with collagen in a new position to decrease the stiffness of the tissue.

There is a lot behind the statements "the muscle is off" or "the muscle is on." Using phrases like this is fine in your patient education, but go deeper in your efforts to understand what these phrases mean.

As the word "psychomotor" in the chapter title implies, we cannot look at motor control from a purely physical perspective. It is the brain that receives sensory input and decides which movement "software" to use in a given situation.

To help our clients fully rehabilitate, we need to retrain their minds and neural systems as well. The following are some of the techniques to help with that.

## PROPRIOCEPTIVE NEUROMUSCULAR FACILITATION

Recent advances in the field of psychomotor control build on the pioneering work of neurophysiologist Herman Kabat did in the 1940s and 1950s. As the basis for creating a new way of restoring function to polio sufferers whose psychomotor control was ravaged by the disease, Kabat used British physiologist Charles Sherrington's Law of Irradiation. The Law of Irradiation states that when one muscle contracts, it recruits other surrounding muscles to increase force production.

He also used Sherrington's complementary idea that agonists and antagonists co-contract in sequence.[150] As I connect some of these concepts, I wonder if this was not early evidence for transmission of force via the deep fascia, as well as the neurological system.

Working with assistants Margaret Knott and Dorothy Voss, Kabat developed a system of neurological rehabilitation that focuses on retraining patients' brains and bodies to enhance motor control and increase the force of muscle contraction.[151]

The use of verbal, proprioceptive, touch-based, and other sensory cues is one of its key components to encourage a client to contract or relax at certain points in a specific range of motion, often in response to resistance.

In addition to using Sherrington's laws, Kabat, Knott, and Voss explored how they might apply other existing physiological principles to neuromotor training. One of these principles was the idea of myostatic stretch reflex, whereby a muscle contracts when quickly lengthened. Another was the inverse stretch reflex, in which pulling on a tendon causes relaxation in the muscle or muscles to which it is attached.

Essentially, Kabat attempted to reeducate patients' brains so that by combining activation and deactivation of agonists and antagonists in various motion sequences and through different planes of motion, they would recover at least some motor control, range of motion, and contractile capacity.

This technique involves all planes of motion, including spiral and diagonal, not just the up-and-down or front-and-back planes dominant in rehab, and is called Proprioceptive Neuromuscular Facilitation (PNF).

While Kabat's initial methods were revolutionary in rehabilitative medicine for sufferers of polio, cerebral palsy, and paralysis from stroke, his assistants brought PNF to the masses. In the 1950s and 1960s, Knott and Voss applied Kabat's PNF system, along with the contributions of Australian nurse Sister Elizabeth Kenney, to other forms of rehabilitation.

This eventually took hold in the athletic training, strength and conditioning, and physical therapy communities as colleges began incorporating PNF in their syllabi for these disciplines.

One of the main reasons for including PNF and its derivatives in the psycho-motor control portion of an athlete's care strategy is to help restore a balance between mobility and stability in movement patterns. This balance is often lost after injury and, in fact, might have contributed to the initial problem.[152]

I often tell athletes they have to earn their mobility. If they lie down to receive passive stretching, it might feel good, but if they do not learn how to use that new range of motion in an upright position, they are going to be in trouble later.

The antagonist of the stretched muscle has to learn to fire within the new range, as does the actual lengthened muscle. If this is not appropriately progressed, we give these clients mobility they do not know how to use or control. That is an injury waiting to happen.

PNF can also help improve coordination and recover the joint and muscular control that can be adversely affected by surgery or by the trauma of an injury. It is also one of the best time-tested ways to get a client to consciously involve the brain in how the body is moving today and should be moving tomorrow.[153]

## MUSCLE ACTIVATION TECHNIQUES

When trying to get an injured athlete back to competitive readiness, we should also consider the work of Greg Roskopf. The MAT® website, *www.muscleactivation.com,* best encapsulates the philosophy of the Roskopf Principle: "Flexibility is a derivative of strength. Muscle tightness is secondary to muscle weakness."

Roskopf devised the MAT system for stimulating muscles so they function at peak efficiency. The starting point of MAT is to assess muscle contraction capabilities. If these are compromised, they will have limited range of motion and, as a result, reduced performance.

In the MAT system, a muscle's health is demonstrated by its ability to efficiently contract, which is vital for normal movement. Any loss of muscle contraction efficiency can manifest itself as a loss of motion, leading to a reduction in physical performance and the development of imbalances and asymmetries that further impede biomechanical function. Such issues can lead to subjective complaints such as soreness or tightness, as well as to diminished physical capabilities.

The goal of MAT is to restore the muscle contraction ability with various force application techniques that make weak muscles stronger and improve range of motion and motor control. Not merely a musculoskeletal approach, MAT also looks at the neuromuscular issues and seeks to remedy them by "reconnecting" the communication between the nerves and muscles.[154]

This brings to mind the "chicken or the egg" debate: *Does muscular weakness compromise mobility or vice versa?*

Roskopf makes a compelling argument for the former. Based on the premise of flexibility deriving from strength, one of the concepts he explores is how to deal with the limiting factor of tight muscles.

Traditionally, the answer has been to stretch or mobilize the muscle perceived as being short or stiff. In this scenario, if you have a client who complains of tight hamstrings, you would mobilize the hamstrings and perhaps, if you were taking a more global approach, the entire posterior chain.

If this is effective, why do clients come back two days later with the same hamstrings tightness?

In the MAT system, the answer would be that they are weak in another muscle group and are asking the hamstrings to work too much as a stabilizer or a mobilizer.

Another option is that the brain has stopped telling the correct muscles to fire at the right time and other muscles—in this case the hamstrings—are being called upon to perform the task. This then shifts the role of other muscles in the motion segment, with prime movers becoming stabilizers and stabilizers becoming synergists.

The body will seek stability where it is lacking. Creating tension in a muscle group is a great way to create artificial stability. If we simply stretch a tight muscle, we might be taking this false yet potentially effective stability away, and, from a stability sense, leaving the client with nothing.

This is an important idea, the concept of firing the antagonist of a tight muscle or muscle group versus stretching the agonist that has lost range of motion or subjectively feels tight. It could be a more effective way of overcoming chronic stiffness and addressing the overactive versus the underactive, and strong versus weak imbalances between opposing muscle groups.

If you can cue an athlete to fire the quads and activate the abdominal muscles, the person may stop "hanging" on the hamstrings, which will in turn lead to that muscle group releasing some of its excess tension.

Again, MAT is recognizing that our physical structures do not act on their own initiatives, but rely on the brain and neural output—which is affected by sensory input—for instructions on what to do, when, and in what sequence.

As we help athletes rebuild their injured bodies, we also have to help them reestablish the neural connections that may have been compromised by injury. Greg Roskopf's MAT practice is one way to accomplish this.

## FUNCTIONAL RANGE CONDITIONING®

Functional Range Conditioning (FRC) is a system of training created by Dr. Andreo Spina. This system works to improve functional mobility and joint health via improved body control. The key concept of the FRC system is the idea of improving the body to handle the movement, not improving the movement itself.

We will discuss concepts of the Dynamic Systems Theory on page 124. In DST, we see the need for the organism to have as many degrees of freedom as possible to express a movement pattern.

A healthier system will have more degrees of freedom to execute a movement. This is a fundamental concept of FRC. If we can improve a body's ability to handle more variables and improve its ability to move with more variability, we will improve movement.

Via a specific progression of movement interventions, the body can begin to express movements of all joints throughout the entire ranges of motion, including its lengthened and shortened ranges.

When each body part is able to achieve this full, active, and useful range of motion, joint health is restored and joint degeneration is minimized. Movement, and therefore function, is improved and pain is mitigated.

FRC is a comprehensive movement intervention. Its concepts fit well within the Motion Segment and Psychomotor Control portions of the *Bridging the Gap* model. Improving and maintaining joint health is key to long-term pain reduction.

## THE POSTURAL RESTORATION INSTITUTE®

The Postural Restoration Institute® (PRI), founded by Ron Hruska, offers another important contribution to psychomotor control training. This training looks at the connection between posture, asymmetrical or imbalanced adaptations, and muscle chains.

One of the key pillars of the PRI school of thought is that the human body is fundamentally asymmetrical and by design, can develop lateralized postural and performance tendencies.

The setup of the organs and components of various systems—including the neural, respiratory, and circulatory systems—are asymmetrical, different in the left and right sides.

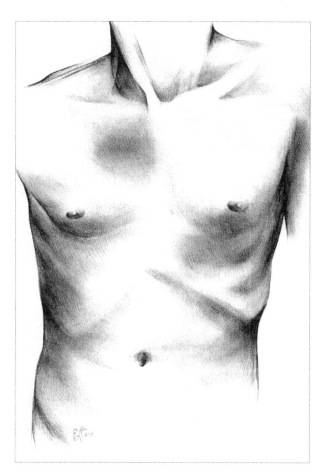

*Illustration by Elizabeth Noble*
*for the Postural Restoration Institute®*
*© 2018 www.posturalrestoration.com*
*Used with permission*

**Figure 5.2—Diaphragm, as Shown by PRI**

*The human body is inherently internally asymmetric. Despite having a symmetrical outward appearance, the organs are singular and located asymmetrically in the body.*

*This asymmetric organ placement and overall design leads to a natural human tendency to shift weight to the right lower body, orient the left half of the pelvis forward, and flare the left lower rib cage, among other compensations.*

*These compensations can be dysfunctional when people are unable to move into and out of these positions at will. These people are no longer able to reposition the diaphragm to the left, derotate the pelvis, or properly shift their center of gravity into the left hemisphere.*

As such, each side of the body is subject to varying postural, positional, and functional demands. In the structure of the torso, we only have one heart, so the chest cavity and surrounding hard and soft structures on the left side are different from those on the right. This shows how anatomical structure can dictate function to some degree.

The setup of the diaphragm is an example that pertains specifically to athlete performance, injury, and rehabilitation. The right dome is larger than the left, with a bigger, thicker, and longer crus on the right side. The right side creates a stronger clockwise lumbar rotation, causing slight right lumbopelvic rotation and increased left thoracic chest expansion as the thorax counter-rotates to the left to stay straight when moving forward. Faulty posturing of the left side of the diaphragm and excessive air in the left chest wall can further contribute to this right lateralization across all body systems.

Since most of us have this anatomy, this is normal human posture. As long as we can move into and out of this position without limitation or faulty compensation, there is no problem. Things can become problematic when we are "stuck" in a pattern and cannot move freely into and out of it.

Certain sports or positions can negate or reverse this "neutral" position. A pitcher who throws thousands of repetitions on one side might eventually develop anticlockwise rotation equally strong or stronger than the capacity to rotate clockwise. There would then be corresponding changes in the reciprocal rotation of the lumbar spine, overcoming the natural functional relationship.

Among unilateral athlete populations, this has a compound effect on stability and mobility in the lumbar and thoracic spine regions. It also affects the muscles and fascia that contribute to the lumbar-pelvic and scapular-shoulder relationships.[155]

The PRI discipline looks at the importance of such correlations between the naturally imbalanced human system and how these influence overall human movement or injury.

The training uses an innovative multi-system approach to changing posture that respects the lateralized tendency of all body systems and has functional implications for all parts of the body. They also suggest exercises and movements that can correct potentially limiting or harmful adaptations that hold back performance and compromise tissue health.

The concepts discussed in PRI are comprehensive and intricate. Thanks to Ron Hruska, MPA, PT, and James Anderson, PT, PRC, for their review of this section. I refer you to *www.posturalrestoration.com* for further information.

## DYNAMIC NEUROMUSCULAR STABILIZATION

The fundamentals of human development tell us that by the time children are three, they are typically able to walk, carry, crawl, and climb. While young children gain the control needed for fine motor skills, their developmental patterns have yet to be corrupted by poor coaching and the eight-hour-a-day sitting that starts in the first grade. You will want to review Kelly Starrett's book *Deskbound* for more on the orthopedic perfect storm created by too much sitting that begins at such an early age.

Once people hit high school or college, they have often subjected their bodies to many years of biomechanical compromises. The functions of an everyday lifestyle—including sports and the postural factors of sitting and standing—start to redefine structure. We become what we behold when it comes to function and structure. This in turn impacts psychomotor control, particularly the ability to stabilize as we move through the world or compete in athletics.

This ability or inability to stabilize is at the core of Dynamic Neuromuscular Stabilization (DNS). Building on the work of the Prague School of Rehabilitation pioneered by Frantisek Vele, Karel Lewit, Vaclav Vojta, and Vladimir Janda, Pavel Kolar has organized a series of movements designed to improve motion-segment function, taking into account the neurological aspects of stabilization. Techniques include manual therapy for reflexive stimulation and three-dimensional stabilizing and strengthening exercises based on the principles of developmental kinesiology.

Dynamic Neuromuscular Stabilization enhances what Kolar and his colleagues call the "Integrated Stabilizing System (ISS)." The area around the spine is comprised of multiple muscles and connective tissues, including the pelvic floor, abdominal wall, diaphragm, intersegmental spinal muscles, and deep neck flexors. The instant before a movement, these tissues should activate in a coordinated way to provide local and global stability.

If one or more component of this functional unit fails to fire, it puts a person at risk not only during sporting activity, but also compromising static loading during sitting and standing.

When just one muscle is not doing its job, the entire stabilizing system becomes less effective, thereby decreasing movement quality. In addition, the body over-recruits other structures in an attempt to add stability, which can result in overuse problems and, in the case of spinal stabilization, possible damage to discs or spinal joints.

To prevent such issues, DNS testing assesses the quality of stabilization to find the weakest link at the root of a stability dysfunction. In the testing, adult function is compared to the "normal" developmental function of an infant.

This developmental kinesiology is then applied to corrective exercises that home in on the ISS. To engage the brain, the ISS is stimulated and activated while the body is in primal developmental positions.[156]

Initially, the clinician provides greater assistance, but as the treatment cycle progresses, the client starts to take more control of the movement patterns.

At first, this is conscious, but once psychomotor control improves, activation of the ISS becomes automatic and subconscious. This stage would ideally coincide with an athlete's return to full practice and competition.[157]

Learning the DNS system can allow a specialist to get to the root of the motor issue by identifying and dealing with the neuromuscular system as a whole.

We see this common theme throughout these interventions: If you change the sensory (afferent) input, you will change the motor (efferent) output.

If you constantly try to alter the motor output without considering the sensory input into the system, you will not get the results you are looking for when addressing movement quality.

## SHIRLEY SAHRMANN MOVEMENT SYSTEM IMPAIRMENT SYNDROMES

Washington University's Program in Physical Therapy is well regarded for good reason. Professor Emerita Shirley Sahrmann and her colleagues were the first to devise and apply a different and highly useful way to look at the role of the neurological system in motor dysfunction: Movement System Impairment Syndromes (MSI).

Sahrmann was the first physical therapist to popularize the evaluation of which muscles and motion segments should be mobile and stable during any particular movement.

She also brought our attention to the consequences if a structure is asked to perform a role in a compensatory pattern that is not its intended job, such as when a stabilizer becomes a prime mover.

The guiding theory of Sahrmann's MSI Syndromes is the idea that biomechanical dysfunction is caused by micro-instability. If there is improper alignment, accessory motions at or between joints—such as roll, spin, or glide—become excessive in one or more directions.

This leads to shearing forces and high-contact pressure within the joints that are not optimally moving and in the surrounding soft tissues, which, if allowed to accumulate over time, can cause macro trauma such as injury, bone deterioration, or damage to muscles, ligaments, or tendons.

Each specific MSI Syndrome is named for the compromised movement alignment or direction at the root of the athlete's warning signs or symptoms, and either removes or decreases these symptoms when corrected.

Sahrmann's MSI method is important to psychomotor control because it allows us to highlight tissue-centric, joint-focused neuromuscular impairments that are either causing the misalignment and micro-instability or making it worse. The MSI Syndrome then provides a guide for treatment, taking into consideration the interplay of various motion segments.[158]

To assess a potential MSI Syndrome, a PT can feel the precision or imprecision of joint motion. If the movement is "incorrect," the PT can manually change it.

We can also address the performance of everyday activities and help fix issues discovered in repeated movements or prolonged postures.[159]

Another key contribution Sahrmann made during her over 50 years in physical therapy education is that it matters how the human body is aligned and moves, and that there are ideals for each movement.

She asserts that there are typically indicators or signs of improper biomechanics and imprecise joint movement that appear before the development of symptoms such as pain or swelling. She teaches that just as biomarkers such as high blood pressure prompt intervention by a professional, so should movement-related red flags.

We can deal with such warning signs through mobility, strengthening, or retraining before everyday activities and exercise ingrain faulty patterns that lead to adaptive changes, and eventually trauma.

It is our job to help our athletes tackle their acute symptoms before they become chronic.[160] Adding Sahrmann's MSI Syndromes to your understanding of neuromuscular control and motor-output improvement would be beneficial for any health care practitioner or sport-performance coach.

Helping each muscle perform its intended job as a prime mover, synergist, or stabilizer will improve the long-term durability of an athlete's system.

## ONE-TUBE STIFFNESS AND SLACK

In addition to giving us the MSI Syndromes, Sahrmann was one of the first PTs to articulate the significance of relative stiffness. In simple terms, this means that the stiffness or slack in a joint, muscle, or motion segment directly influences the tone of structures farther up or down the kinetic chain.[161]

In recent presentations, I used this idea in relation to the tube that runs from the mouth, down the esophagus, into the gut, and all the way to the anus, referencing the stiffness and slack of the surrounding tissues at different points along the line.

If we see people who have difficulty breathing from the diaphragm, have

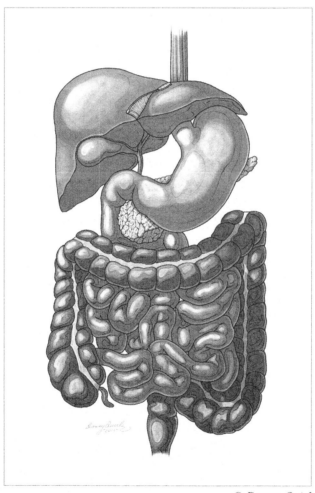

© Danny Quirk

**Figure 5.3—Creating Homeostasis**

*There is one long tube from the mouth to the anus. Tension in one part of this tube will affect the others. When someone presents with "neck tension" in the top of the tube, in order to maintain homeostasis in the tube, it must slacken part of it—the "core"—and the core becomes flaccid.*

*We focus on trying to decrease tension at the neck, but don't try to increase the tension at the core. We need to look at this area as one unit.*

upper-quarter stiffness that results in chronically sore upper traps or neck pain, or who struggle with GERD, we typically do not think about the stiffness or laxity in the entire system, and instead focus on local issues and solutions. However, per the relative stiffness theory, when tight in the upper back and neck, there must be slack elsewhere in the system where it does not belong.

When evaluating clients who suffer from symptoms farther along this tube, I often find they are not creating primary stability; there is too much slack in the centrally located base of support. A body looks to somewhere else up the tube—the neck, for example, is a common site of tension—to create artificial stiffness, as it will always find stability.[162]

If we can get people to consciously reengage the abdominals and eventually get them to autonomously create stability, the stiffness in other areas may be reduced, as well as possibly relieving the symptoms.

Another way to look at this is through a mobility lens. Increasing hip mobility allows us to squat deeper and maybe stay in this position for different activities during the day, whether using the toilet, gardening, or practicing yoga.

When we squat deeply, the thighs push into the belly and the belly pushes back, creating intra-abdominal pressure. In creating pressure, we are creating stiffness or stability at the trunk. If we can create stability in the trunk, the upper traps or neck region can relax, as the "tube" searches for balanced

tension throughout its length. In essence, improving hip mobility might help decrease neck stiffness.

This is another example of the brain telling the body how best to position itself. It also demonstrates that we cannot merely look at a single motion segment as the site of a client's symptoms when trying to get past the 70–80 percent recovery sticking point many encounter.

## CLINICAL PEARL

If one end of the system is tight, the other end is going to be slack. You can't "release" one end without "stabilizing" the other. Decreasing neck tension goes hand in hand with core stabilization.

## FUNCTIONAL MOVEMENT SCREEN AND SELECTIVE FUNCTIONAL MOVEMENT ASSESSMENT

One of the reasons for including the Functional Movement Screen (FMS) and the Selective Functional Movement Assessment (SFMA) in this section as well as in the previous chapter is that Gray Cook and company recognize that the body's function—the "motor" part—is governed by the mind's direction—the "psycho" component. As Cook has said, "Your brain is too smart to allow you to have full horsepower in a bad body position. It is called muscle inhibition."

In the three states that govern movement pattern selection and quality—input, processing, and output—we often overlook the idea that motor control and mobility problems can be caused by a brain-based "processing" error.

The FMS and SFMA assessments give us a relatively simple and standardized way of finding faulty output and working backward to address the processing and input errors.

Once an athlete's weak point has been uncovered by the FMS or SFMA, we can use corrective exercises to assist in the movement expression. These scaled-back exercises are designed to eliminate the chance to compensate. The regressed exercises break down movements into basic components to rewire how the brain chooses, sequences, and coordinates motor patterns.

If an athlete is having a psychomotor problem during rehabilitation that has led to a coordination issue between upper- and lower-body motion, you might assign crawling, half-kneeling, and quadruped drills to rebuild the patterning from the ground up—literally.

If a client is having trouble performing a loaded barbell squat, you could unload the exercise and start with bodyweight or air squats, or maybe going from the top to bottom or bottom to top positions.[163]

You could also use equipment, such as a plyo box, to suggest a box squat variation as you help the athlete improve motor control and mobility. Then, when able to demonstrate competence in the most basic, unloaded version of a movement, you could add a systemic stressor like load, speed, or unilateral balance, such as a one-leg or pistol squat.

Sometimes simply loading a movement pattern will help clean up its faults. Taking away an athlete's ability to compensate in a bilateral task by turning it into a unilateral task can engage the motion segment you need to enhance. Progressions and regressions are not always cut and dry…nor are they linear.

What might be a progression for one athlete could be a regression for another, based on the movement pattern and the person's needs, as well as the response to verbal or tactile cues. If you are not getting the movement pattern you want, you will have to change the stimulus.

## PILATES

Pilates-based activities and theories can be helpful techniques for the clinician or performance coach, particularly when trying to reestablish psychomotor control in an athlete who is moving through the bridging-the-gap process.

While you would not use it to build power as in Olympic lifting or explosiveness as you might with plyometrics, Joseph Pilates's system has its place in the rehabilitation spectrum, particularly when it comes to enhancing psychomotor control.[164]

When this German immigrant came to America in 1925 and started popularizing his transformative training methods out of his New York studio, his system did not bear his name. Perhaps this is because of his modesty, but the more likely explanation is that Pilates believed his work was better described in a way that honored the brain-body connection he emphasized.

This is why Pilates first dubbed it "Contrology," implying that it was the mind that led to the heightened degree of motor control his exercise program cultivated. Pilates stated that, "It is the mind itself that controls the body," his variation on a favorite saying of German philosopher Friedrich von Schiller.[165]

One of the reasons the Pilates system is useful in bringing clients back to competition readiness is that it is scalable. It is not until an athlete can master a basic position in an unloaded state that a Pilates trainer will add resistance of some kind to challenge positional integrity.

If you have an athlete who is experiencing pain or expressing limited range of motion in a motion segment, Pilates movements can be scaled, using equipment with springs to assist difficult movement patterns to take into account the limitation. Once having moved toward recovery, resistance and loading with equipment like the Reformer can be introduced to further enhance psychomotor control.

Spine-first stabilization is another thing to like about the Pilates method. As he put it, "A man is as young as his spinal column." If we are thinking about health—as we should—we need to consider the spine as essential to the survival of the human organism.

When it comes to posture, the main purpose of organizing the trunk—and all that core stability work we put our clients through—is not for its own sake, but to protect the spinal cord, which is the central line of communication between the brain and body.

If an athlete is having trouble achieving and maintaining stability in the torso, you would do well to look to Pilates to improve positioning.[166]

This primary stability will make it easier to create stiffness in other motion segments in the body.

Breathing is the third factor that should endear Pilates to any professional seeking to improve an athlete's psychomotor control. While its founder was unwavering about the neurological and physical benefits his methodology offered, he was very clear about the necessary foundation for a healthy life, saying, "Above all, learn how to breathe correctly."

Yoga, which we will discuss in the chapter on somatosensory control beginning on page 131, gets all the press when it comes to the link between breathing and body control, yet it is just as central in Pilates. This is one more reason to bring a certified Pilates instructor into your professional circle to advance your clients' journey back to full capacity.[167]

## SUMMARY

Psychomotor control is all about the right muscle firing at the right time. It ensures that all elements of the system are doing their proper jobs when it comes to movement.

Agonists should be the prime movers for specific movements; antagonists should resist those movements. Then, synergists should assist the movements.

Stabilizers should stabilize the body so force can be developed to create the movement.

When stabilizers become movers and prime movers become synergists, the body gets angry and pain ensues.

There is a huge neurological impact on movement, which we will discuss shortly. Sensory input will affect motor output.

Therefore, if motor output is faulty, altering sensory input is often required to fix it.

# CHAPTER SIX
## THE BIOPSYCHOSOCIAL MODEL

George Engel was a psychiatrist credited for his work in psychiatry, specifically in creating what we know as the biopsychosocial model of health care.[168] The biopsychosocial model includes the typical biomedical model of health care and includes the psychological, social, and behavioral aspects of medicine that significantly influence the physical body and its ability to repair.

We discussed the individuality of pain earlier beginning on page 42; however, these concepts can be applied to other aspects of health care.

For example, as health care and performance specialists, we like to believe that everyone wants to feel better, get better, and get back out onto the field. I cannot tell you how many people say, "Wow, you work with professional athletes? That must be so great, always getting to work with people who are so motivated to get better." This might be expected, but it is not always the case.

There is a significant role of psychology, social pressures, and mindset during rehabilitation. If you do not monitor and address these elements, the things you learn in this book will not be helpful.

Virtually none of the physical things we are discussing can happen if people have the mindset that it may not be in their best interest to get better, to let go of the injury and pain, and move forward in their lives.

Let us take, for example, a baseball player who is injured. The rehab is going well, and the person is getting ready to return to the field. However, the player who was brought up to take the place of the injured teammate is also doing well. Everyone from the fans to management is happy with this new player's performance and the excitement he brings to the field every day.

What happens if the injured player gets better and then does not get returned to his spot on the roster? How would it feel if the injured athlete is not playing because the new player is better than he is, not because he is hurt?

Ego will subconsciously kick in to tell us it is better to be hurt than to be a lesser player than another who has taken the spot—stay hurt. If you are injured, they cannot expect you to play. For no apparent physical reason, the pain does not ease fully and the injured player might not make your timeline goals. The athlete just is not getting better.

Letting go of pain has consequences, not all of which are positive. When people are in pain or injured, they cannot be held responsible for everything that might be required of them in daily life.

Taking care of the household, the kids, the job, and the pets all become overwhelming when in an injured state.

If people have pain or an injury, asking for help is a reasonable thing to do. When someone is not injured, asking for help could be perceived as a weakness— the inability to keep everything together and do it all.

This does not happen all the time. The point is, for a patient, there needs to be value in getting better. Sometimes getting better does not hold the value we expect it would.

There are often psychological components of the rehab process you may not feel comfortable with or qualified to handle. You do not have to personally deal with these aspects of recovery, but if you are working with people who are trying to bridge the gap from rehab to performance, you need to recognize that these psychological issues exist and build a referral source who can help you navigate them.

Broaching the subject of a psychological component to pain and injury can be difficult for many health care and strength and conditioning professionals. It is a subject you need to address carefully and with sensitivity.

Simply asking athletes how they are holding up during the rehab process may kick start a conversation. Talking to them about how they are feeling in general— not physically, but generally— may be the catalyst to a deeper conversation. Acknowledging that the rehab

process is long and difficult and seeing how they respond can also begin this conversation.

The next section describes how different professionals in the bridging-the-gap continuum can assist an athlete with the psychological piece of the rehabilitation puzzle. We can do a lot to support the biopsychosocial model, and there are signs and symptoms to recognize when an athlete might need professional help beyond your scope.

One of the great things about working in a professional sport team is the uninhibited access the athletes have to many professionals. It is very easy for one of the athletic trainers or physical therapists to talk with the sport psychologist when an athlete is exhibiting concerning signs and symptoms. The sport psychologist could then nonchalantly begin talking with athlete, offering services in a benign way.

When you do not work in this setting, it is important to bring up the subject of professional help in a delicate manner. Asking athletes how they are doing may be enough opportunity for you to say, "If you want to talk to someone, we have this person available."

If an athlete is exhibiting signs that concern you, being direct in saying you are concerned and want the person to speak to someone may be the best route.

Do not allow your uncomfortable feelings about this subject prevent you from suggesting your athletes get the help they need.

## THE PSYCHOLOGY AND MINDSET OF INJURY

An injury comes with a set of emotions. Anger, sadness, fear, irritability, changes in appetite, or behavior have all been associated with injury.[169] These emotions are normal and we should acknowledge them. However, at times these emotions can get overwhelming and hinder an athlete's ability to move forward in the rehab process toward a productive stage of injury management.

You should call in a mental health professional who deals with sport-performance or injury-related issues if you notice significant behavioral changes, such as extreme sadness or anger, or there are notable appetite changes showing up as drastic increases or decreases in weight, or the athlete begins unhealthy behaviors such as binging and purging.

Having a person with these credentials on speed dial is vital to the bridging-the-gap team you are creating for your recovering athletes.

Each health care professional and performance specialist plays a role in the recovery of an injured athlete. Athletic trainers who use short-term goals and a variety of rehab exercises have been shown to mentally help injured athletes.[170] Physical therapists have been successful with tools such as behavioral outcome measures and the use of mental imagery during the rehab process.ʼ

Athletes appreciate strength coaches who listen without giving advice or being judgmental, as well as those who notice when an athlete works hard during the rehab process.[171,172]

Finally, skill and sport coaches can be helpful in keeping an athlete involved in team activities and in helping to find a support person, such as a former athlete who has previously gone through a similar recovery progression.[173]

Every professional along the way can have a significant impact in the mental health of a rehabilitating athlete. It is no single person's job to address or monitor an athlete's mental health. Any person in the bridging-the-gap continuum may notice subtle behavior changes in their area that another professional might not see.

Great inter-staff communication is vital for helping an injured athlete get back to the field to play.

## BRAIN MEETS BODY: THE EMOTIONAL AND PSYCHOLOGICAL LOAD OF PAIN

To continue this line of thinking, when we think about pain, we often consider the physical sensation. However, as we cannot separate a body from its brain, we also need to factor in the emotional and psychological impacts that an injury and being in pain has on our clients.

For an athlete who has suffered an identifiable event like an ankle injury while playing a sport, we cannot just rehab the body so the person can return to active status—we also need to help get the mind right.

An athlete must overcome fear of repeating the specific action and getting hurt again. A surfer who suffered a bad wipeout that tore a shoulder labrum will be wary about dropping into a wave even when physically able to get back in the water.

There is another component that can slow an athlete's recovery called "kinesiophobia"—the fear of movement that creates pain. The movement doesn't even need to be performed. Simply the thought of performing that movement can cause enough anxiety that the athlete will struggle with return-to-play progressions.

Athletes recognize the sports-medicine professional's involvement in the psychological aspect of an injury. These professionals identify simple things like setting attainable goals and holding athletes accountable through the rehab process, including not allowing missed sessions, and using subtle motivation as helpful interventions during recovery from injury.[174]

Athletes also acknowledge that support from their strength and conditioning coaches is valuable during the rehab process. These people who listen without giving advice or judgment, called "listening support," and those who view the world as the athlete does, known as "reality confirmation," have been demonstrated to be valuable psychosocial support.[175]

Other ways of contributing include appreciating and verbalizing that the athlete is working hard, keeping the athlete challenged and engaged, and "keeping it real." These techniques have all been shown to be valuable as patients work through the rehab process.[176]

If these do not suffice, it might then be time to involve a sports psychologist or mental conditioning coach.

At a basic level, you can help your athletes by talking them through their fears and reassuring that they are not on this journey alone. Ensuring that athletes feel like they have a support team and that they are not alone is vital to a healthy mind and, thus, a healthy body. Often, simply listening to the fears and concerns of our clients can have a huge impact on their psychological health when working through the rehabilitative process.

Without making guarantees, our goal is to have the athletes return bigger, faster, or stronger than their pre-injury state. Our aim is not only to rehabilitate an injury, but also to return each client to athletics more biomechanically sound than before the incident.

We can use this time in rehab to address long-term biomechanical dysfunctions that may have been present but that perhaps were not addressed earlier due to a lack of time between competitive events. This is now the time to let the current injury heal while working on things that could have possibly contributed outside of the general physics that were brought to bear at the time of injury.

Being in pain for a long time does not just lead to short-term changes; it can actually cause rewiring in multiple areas of the brain.

In a study published in *Neuroscience Behavior Review*, Laura Simon, Igor Elman and David Borsook state that "Experiencing pain can trigger a cascade of neurological events—initially sensory—that lead to an altered psychological state; and prior psychological states can confer a heightened risk for pain chronicity due to processes such as cross sensitization, where exposure to stress in the past results in greater sensitivity to other seemingly unrelated stimuli."[177]

What Simon and her colleagues are saying is that a single pain event can change our psychology, and that the brain then primes people to overreact or go into a chronic pain state when next exposed to a pain stimulus. In addition, the changes that pain prompts in one area of brain function, such as cognition, can have a knock-on negative effect on others—like memory. This is why chronic pain is considered to be its own pathology outside of any lingering physical issues an injury might create.

In the study, they identified multiple parts of the brain affected by the stress load of chronic pain, including the cerebellum, basal ganglia, and prefrontal cortex. Along with the motor cortex, these are the primary brain regions responsible for selecting and implementing movement patterns.

An athlete who has been suffering from chronic pain may have experienced alterations in the circuitry in these areas,

which in turn impacts the ability to perform athletic skills.

This is why the player you are trying to get back on the field might need help with relearning basic skills like running and more advanced proficiencies related to a specific sport or position.[178]

People who are fearful of returning to normal movements have developed a "fear avoidance pattern of movement." They will literally avoid any movement they fear will cause further damage. This threat of damage does not even have to be real. No matter how it appears to us, it is realistic to the patient, and therefore, the person will avoid these movements at all costs.

Implementing things like the Fear Avoidance Belief Questionnaire,[179] which you can easily find via a Google search, can be helpful in determining a client's fear of movement activities.

Patient-reported outcome measures (PROMs) are status reports about the patient's health that come directly from the patient, without interpretation by a clinician. In PROMs, patients fill out a questionnaire reporting how they feel, what functional measures and improvements they have experienced, and what continues to cause them trouble.

PROMs are extremely valuable in gaining insight on patients' opinions of their recovery status, which is what matters when returning from an injury.

These can also help as you employ techniques like goal setting during the rehab process. You and the client both know that the ultimate aim is to return to full function in playing the sport. Nevertheless, if you set smaller incremental goals along the way, it will give the athlete something to focus on other than pain.[180]

When people are active participants in their care and understand the timelines set forth for short-term goal achievement, it helps shed the victim mentality that can develop in people who are struggling with pain.

## MEDITATION

Meditation is another technique many people use to deal with the stresses of injury and recovery. People define meditation in many ways,[181] making it difficult to develop a general program dealing with the topic. Meditation is an individual practice that can range from religious and spiritual to simply being a way to relax.

However you choose to define mediation for the people you work with, it is worth having a few specific ideas you can easily implement.

Many physiological and psychological benefits have been shown with a breath-based meditation program.[182] Specifically, a yogic breath program can be helpful. Deep, slow, rhythmic breathing can reduce stress and anxiety and help balance the autonomic nervous system.[183]

Breath-based meditation has also been shown as helpful in modulating physical and emotional overload, and may be useful in human performance in times of acute or chronic stress.[184]

If an athlete is open to the idea, breath-based meditation may be a great way to start, as it connects something that is not tangible—the concepts of meditation—to something very tangible...breathing. As it stimulates the autonomic nervous system, it decreases the effects of depression, stress, and anxiety, all of which often accompany injury.[185]

You can also use imagery as a form of meditation. Having an athlete sit quietly and visualize the desired outcome can have positive benefits.

It can be helpful to use some of the visualization techniques Dr. Jim Afremow introduces in his excellent book *The Champion's Comeback*, which teaches an injured athlete how to mentally rehearse a successful return to the court, field, or pitch. This book is worth your review.

Visualization can create a stronger positive bond between what the mind pictures the body doing and what the athlete physically does. This can help replace negative pain-related fear with a positive expectation of success.[186]

Imagery should use all five senses to be truly effective; simply visualizing what might happen may not be enough. Having the athlete also focus on other sensations—the roar of the crowd, the smell of the grass, the taste of their gum, and the feel of the bat in hand—is likely to make the imaging more tangible, thus making the exercise more effective.

## RECOVERY AND REGENERATION STRATEGIES

Recovery is the overall process by which an athlete recuperates from a physical stress and the time it takes to do so while not overstressing the system. Regeneration strategies are as those practices we do to help the recovery process as a whole.

These regeneration strategies can be active or passive. Some are more tried and tested than others; however, every person is different and it is worth trying different modalities to see what works best for each athlete.

Techniques such a massage, contrast bath, cold tub, cryochambers, intermittent compression pumps, and more have all been used, tested, supported, and refuted in the literature. First, do no harm with these modalities. If one of these makes an athlete "feel better," there is value in that; whether that value is mental or physical is up for debate. The placebo effect is strong and the mental benefit can be just as if not more powerful than the physiological benefit.

Massages are a key to the recovery and regeneration processes. There are many documented benefits to having someone physically work on a body's soft tissues.[187,188,189] Depending on the type of massage, directed tissue work can be performed for a prolonged period on a given day, versus 10–15 minutes on a different day.

This physical tissue manipulation may be needed to assist in strengthening scar tissue and in scar maturation. This type of massage is far from relaxing; it can be quite painful. A more peaceful, light touch soft-tissue massage works well for stress management and relaxation. It all depends on what the athlete needs at the time.

A contrast bath is a regeneration technique commonly used in athletics. Hot tubs and cold tubs are in professional athletic training rooms worldwide, as well as in most colleges and even in some high schools.

It is common to use either a cold tub or a contrast bath at some point during the week; however, do we really know what they do?

A systematic review by Breger Stanton et al in 2009[190] looked at 28 research studies on contrast baths from 1938 to 2008 and found the range of conditions and protocols made it difficult to form a conclusive opinion on its use. There were no definitive correlations to functional outcomes or swelling control, although there is some evidence for increasing skin temperature and superficial blood flow.

Higgins et al[191] found limited changes in performance scores post contrast or ice bath. While the use of contrast or ice baths are prevalent in our sports culture, limited physical benefits have been noted. However, mental or placebo effects may be strong, which is what continues to drive their use.

Intermittent compression devices are another common modality used for recovery and regeneration. Although there is some athlete perception and self-reported decrease in muscle soreness, minimal objective measurements of improved performance or recovery have been found.[192,193,194]

The lack of objective improvements in recovery or performance do not negate the use of intermittent compression devices in recovery and regeneration plans, given the patient-reported outcome of "feeling better" after its use.

Cryochambers—whole-body cryotherapy—are the newest additions to many sports-performance and recovery centers. An athlete will enter a chamber cooled by nitrogen or other mechanisms to around minus 140 degrees Celsius and will remain in the chamber for no longer than three minutes. This is either a walk-in chamber or one where the body is enclosed, but the head is out. Body mass index influences its ability to cool tissue.

While many benefits and changes have been shown with its use—including changes to core body temperature, alterations in metabolism, hematological responses, inflammatory markers, endocrine responses, muscle, sports performance recovery, and pain[195]—whole-body cryotherapy is controversial due to its contraindications and potential for injury if there is sweat or water anywhere on the body. Whole-body cryotherapy should be used with caution for rehabilitation, and only by a trained professional.

Patient perception is strong and extremely valuable when talking about recovery and regeneration techniques.

If athletes think they feel better, there is significant value in its continued use in sports-performance recovery.

Placebo may not be a good thing when reading research or when in a lab; however, clinically, placebo is a powerful element, and in my opinion is useful when it comes to what an athlete chooses to use to feel better.

Just because placebo may not be statistically significant in a lab, it can be clinically significant in the real world.

We as clinicians and coaches must recognize the limitation of our devices. We should acknowledge that these interventions may work, just not for the reasons we think.

## SLEEP

Sleep is one of the most powerful of recovery strategies, and has been discussed more in recent years. Lack of sleep has been linked to everything from obesity, impulse control, blood pressure changes, heart disease, mood disturbances, cancer, and more.

For the rehabilitating athlete, sleep is just as important, if not more, than other therapeutic interventions we might use. Physiological processes affecting physical health and the ability to heal will be negatively impacted if an athlete who is trying to bridge the gap from rehab to performance is not experiencing quality sleep.

Sleep, like breathing, is not optional.

During my time in Major League Baseball, I had the pleasure of working with Dr. Chris Winter and was recently thrilled to receive a copy of his new book *The Sleep Solution*. I refer you to it for a comprehensive look at this powerful recovery tool.

If this is not your area of expertise, start your study now. Use books like Dr. Winter's to improve your knowledge on the subject and to help your athletes implement simple and effective strategies to improve their sleep habits.

## NUTRITION

Quality nutrition is another aspect of recovery we cannot ignore. I have been lucky in my career to always have a nutritionist within walking distance of my office. In fact, during my time at EXOS, we found nutrition to be so important for the rehabilitating athlete that we began having the nutritionist meet with every rehab client who walked through the door.

Regeneration and the healing of tissue is hard work on the body. Caloric expenditure must be analyzed and managed by a professional to avoid unwanted weight loss or gain during the rehab process. It is key to limiting pro-inflammatory foods along with increasing anti-inflammatory foods.

Proper hydration is required for the cellular processes of healing. Helping our athletes implement simple strategies to keep them on track during the bridging-the-gap process is essential for compliance.

Working with a professional with significant understanding of this subject is so important for the rehabilitating athlete. It is a complicated topic that is beyond the scope of this text to comprehensively tackle.

Please seek more information from the resources in Appendix Nine and work with knowledgeable professionals who can help guide you toward the information your clients need.

## REGENERATION DAYS

Regeneration days are essential as the athlete begins to transition toward the performance side of the continuum. Athletes cannot simply work themselves back to the field. They must allow the body time to adapt to stresses placed on the system, or their bodies will break down due to overloading. This is the concept of super compensation, which we will discuss in Chapter Nine.

Regeneration days are planned active days of rest. Mentally, this helps the athlete prepare for the week ahead. An athlete is more likely to take a scheduled day of active rest knowing it is a planned day versus showing up to the facility one day and hearing, "You have the day off."

Athletes like to be in control and they like to have control of their schedules. When they know an active day of rest is planned in advance, compliance is higher and they recognize it as part of the process versus you perhaps not wanting to work with them that day.

An active regeneration day can take many forms. It can involve a pool workout, where all the movements you have been working on during the week are now done in an unloaded state in the water. It might consist of a game of Frisbee, a hike, or bike ride. It can be any activity that gives athletes a day away from the confines of the gym or clinic, but keeps them active.

A more passive regeneration day might consist of a massage, relaxing with family, or watching a movie. This includes anything that gets their minds off the active work and assists in destressing the brain, and therefore the body.

## SUMMARY

There is much more to bridging the gap from rehab to performance than the physical components we discuss in this book. In fact, the mental component may play a larger role in the overall process of returning to play.

It is essential to be aware of the psychological issues that come along with injury and are prepared to deal with them within your scope of practice.

Referring to a mental health care professional at any point in the process is key for successful outcomes with an athlete who is struggling.

Good recovery and regeneration strategies must be implemented in order for the athletes to adapt to physical stresses. Modalities can be helpful in the process, and sleep, nutrition, and hydration are key components in the bridging-the-gap process.

# CHAPTER SEVEN
## SOMATOSENSORY CONTROL

As strength coaches, personal trainers, and clinicians, we like the motor system end of things. We can see it in action. It is tangible. The "sensory" part of the somatosensory system is harder to reckon with. You cannot touch balance or proprioception; these are conceptual.

Yet they are no less important than the musculoskeletal system when it comes to recovery and rehabilitation, and are in fact indivisible from it. We cannot expect to move effectively, efficiently, or sustainably unless the senses are giving us the context to do so.

According to Dr. Patrick Dougherty from MD Anderson Cancer Center:

> *"The somatosensory systems inform us about objects in our external environment through touch (i.e., physical contact with skin) and about the position and movement of our body parts (proprioception) through the stimulation of muscles and joints.*

> *"The somatosensory systems also monitor the temperature of the body, external objects, and environment, and provide information about painful, itchy, and tickling stimuli."* [196]

In other words, the somatosensory system deals with the sensory aspect of the sensorimotor system (SMS).

The sensorimotor system encompasses all of the sensory input, motor output, central processing, and the integration of these components during movement.[197]

From a biomechanical and kinesthetic standpoint, we could not have a motor system without a sensory system. The input gives us the output. Bad input equals bad output.

If we continually type the wrong command into the computer, we get the wrong output every time. We have to give the computer the correct instructions for it to work properly. The same goes for the body. With altered information coming in, the motor response will be faulty or, at best, inefficient.

Balance, postural sway, reflexes, and proprioceptive awareness are all considerations when we are dealing with the somatosensory system.

We can define somatosensory control as the sensory input focus on the SMS processes. In fact, most of the material discussed in this book is dependent upon and related to the SMS. Sensory input will affect motor output.

I often pull from my experiences with DNS, PRI, yoga, and Pilates to assist a client's balance, proprioception, and reflexive responses. In this chapter, we will explore how various sensory manipulations like visual and vestibular can be used to improve somatosensory control as athletes continue the journey to back to competition.

## THE DYNAMIC SYSTEMS THEORY

The Dynamic Systems Theory (DST) gives us a framework for which we can assess and treat, truly creating "functional training" programs for our clients. The DST states that the sensorimotor system of a given person is dependent upon the health or dis-ease of the organism, the task, and the environment in which the task is being executed.

These three things—the task, the organism, and the environment in which the movement is being performed—will all dictate which movement pattern is selected by the patient.

Let us look at these in more detail.

**Organism constraints:** *A healthy organism can use multiple degrees of freedom to complete a task.*

The concept of functional variability tells us there are many ways for a person to complete a task. In general, the SMS will organize itself in a way that is simple for the nervous system or conserves the overall energy of the organism.

For example, as you are reading this, reach up and touch your nose. Did you use your right hand or left hand? Which finger did you use? Did you bring your arm up and round your neck or did you bend your elbow to raise your arm to touch your nose?

There are multiple ways for the SMS to execute this goal of "touch your nose." The SMS probably took the easiest way it knew how: Most of us use our dominant hand and the index finger we typically use to point to things. The SMS has developed an efficient way of doing such tasks. There is no "wrong" way to touch your nose. You most likely did it in the simplest, most efficient way you knew.

Now, if you had a broken dominant arm in a cast, you could not use that arm. The organism now has fewer degrees of freedom from which to choose to perform the movement. It can only use the non-dominant arm.

Dis-ease of a system due to injury, neurological deficit, or pain will all diminish the degrees of freedom the SMS has to perform a task. In this way, the SMS has less functional variability.

When manipulating the organism within the DST, we can have the organism close both eyes or turn the head, track a moving object, perform a cognitive task while moving, or do an unrelated upper-extremity activity while performing a lower-body movement.

Manipulating the organism to change the degrees of available freedom allows us to provide our clients with functional variability.

This is something most athletes need as they return to sport, as there are multiple things to think about and do in addition to just running forward.

**Task constraints:** *The task we are asking the person to perform can have varying degrees of difficulty.*

Manipulating the task is often the most common way practitioners change what is being done from a rehab or performance standpoint.

For example, when we ask people to squat, they can do it in a variety of ways. They can squat on two legs, squat on one leg, front squat, back squat, goblet squat…the list goes on and on.

Manipulating the task is an essential component to the DST, but we need to remember it is only one component.

Manipulating the task takes into account a person's base of support and center of gravity. Typically, we can make a task harder by decreasing the base of support—such as moving from two legs to one leg—or altering the center of gravity by bringing them from the ground to standing, to holding something overhead or out in front. Progressions and regressions of a task often take into account both of these variables.

**Environment constraints:** *If we ask a person to bring a package across the room, it may be a simple, predictable task.*

The person may pick up the box, turn around, walk across the room, and put the package down. However, if we ask again, but turn on loud music, put obstacles in the way, and have other people running around in the path, this becomes an unpredictable environment. The SMS now has to make decisions to safely perform the task.

We can manipulate the environment in several ways. We often think about eyes closed versus eyes open, which is an organism constraint, but what about varying degrees of light?

Think about a day game versus a night game in baseball. During the day, people talk about shadows that go across the field. The players' eyes remain open, but the light will alter what they see and when they see it.

Imagine practicing hitting in your backyard versus hitting in front of 50,000 people screaming and yelling, sometimes directly at you.

Think about obstacles that may be in the way when completing a task. Running from first to second seems pretty direct, but sometimes a middle infielder covering the base will be in the way. The task of running to second just got more difficult because of the change in environment.

Consider running a marathon. If you trained in 60-degree weather the entire time you prepared, on a 60-degree event day, you would know exactly how much and how often you needed to drink to stay hydrated, what you needed to eat for energy, and what you needed to do to recover.

If you get to the event and it is 90 degrees, all your training may be out the window. You may be running the same distance, along the same route, but the environment is very different. Your time may be slower than you expect; your hydration needs will change and your post-race recovery will be extremely different.

The changed environment made your task a lot more difficult.

---

## CLINICAL PEARL

### Dynamic Systems Theory IS functional training

- **Affect the organism**—increase the degrees of freedom the organism has to complete the task

- **Alter the task**—manipulate the base of support or center of gravity

- **Change the environment**—alter the sights, sounds, or surface of training

---

## PROVIDING A FRAMEWORK OF FUNCTIONAL TRAINING

You can see how the Dynamic Systems Theory can provide a framework of "functional training." The organism constraints will limit the number of degrees of freedom available to perform a task, and the environment can significantly impact the way the task is performed. We can also make the task more difficult by altering the base of support or center of gravity.

Using principles from the DST can provide you with a systematic way to challenge the SMS. As discussed, task manipulation is often the easiest and most common way for a practitioner to progress an exercise program.

However, if all we do is change the task, we are missing out on two key elements of the DST.

The next time you have the opportunity to experiment with programming, try not changing the task for two weeks. Instead, during week one, alter the organism.

For example, if you have your clients performing a squat—the task—you can manipulate the organism by having them squat while looking left and right.

Quite frankly, that is most likely how they would perform the task anyway; rarely do people squat to the ground with perfect form while looking straight ahead. Chances are, they might be talking to someone, looking one direction, squatting down, maybe looking down to pick up an object, and then return to standing.

Another example would be to have them take their shoes off, or have them perform a cognitive task as they squat—have them to count to 100 in threes.

Does their form change? Have them track a swinging ball while performing the squat—does eye movement alter their execution of the task?

Next, alter the environment. Have the person perform the task with music blaring, or perhaps without it if music is normal, with the lights off—be safe—or outside, on a balance beam, on foam, or in sand.

How does manipulating the environment change the execution?

When you begin to consider manipulating more than just the task, you will find week's worth of progressions without ever changing the exercise.

This is the framework for "functional training:" giving the organism as many degrees of freedom possible to perform any task, in any given environment.

---

### CLINICAL PEARL

**Functional training**—giving the organism as many degrees of freedom possible to perform any task, in any given environment

---

## THE VISUAL SYSTEM: WHAT YOU SEE IMPACTS HOW YOU MOVE

Our eyes are one way the motor system receives feedback. We cannot ignore the importance of touch or hearing in providing context that helps us decide which movement patterns to access and deploy. However, just two and eight percent, respectively, of the brain's sensory neurons are devoted to these, while 30 percent deal exclusively with input from the visual system.[198]

Altering the visual system in a way that is meaningful can be a great way to manipulate organism constraints. The most common constraint a clinician or coach will do is to have people close their eyes. This is a fine constraint manipulation, but how realistic is that to sport? Usually the athletes' eyes will be open and they will not be looking straight ahead on a fixed point.

Consider, for example, standing on a single leg. You can have people stand on one leg and close their eyes.

Alternatively, you could have them stand on one leg, keep their heads straight forward, and have their eyes follow a moving ball on a string dangling in front of them.

You could have them keep their heads straight and look up and to the left or right, focusing on something in their peripheral vision while they perform the task. You could use glasses that prevent the use of peripheral vision. You can have them track a moving object with just their eyes or with the entire head while performing a task.

There are multiple ways to alter vision, more than just having the eyes open or closed. These other considerations are often more specific to what an athlete would be doing on the field. Consider the addition of sunglasses, helmets, or tinted contacts to your rehab progressions if your athletes use these devices in their sport.

## THE VESTIBULAR SYSTEM: BALANCE IN MOTION

When athletes are coming back from an injury, balance and proprioception are often the biggest challenges—the recognition of where they are and how they are moving through the environment.

They also often struggle with maintaining equilibrium. To restore this in the past, we mistakenly had them spend a lot of time on balls and balance boards—tippy surfaces we thought would help restore reactive balance.

If we consider most sports, the ground itself is not moving or tilting unless we are talking about water and some winter sports. Rather, the athlete is moving over the ground. The ground is not unstable; it is uneven. This is why we have athletes work on restoring the vestibular input and control on a stable terrain.

The TerraSensa® is a useful complement to this, particularly if conditions prevent us from getting the athlete outside, because it features bumps and divots that simulate variable topography.

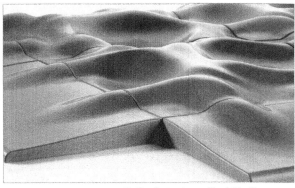

© *Ludwig Artzt GmbH, Germany*

**Photo 7.1—TerraSensa**

*Altering the surface upon which a movement is performed is a common practice among practitioners.*

*The typical progression is to place someone on an unstable surface, such as a foam pad or half ball.*

*However, rarely will an athlete be in a position needing to manage an unstable surface—what will most likely be encountered is an uneven surface.*

*Using a product like the TerraSensa can give the practitioner a way to do this indoors, challenging the client in a more safe and controlled manner than outside on a field.*

Having an athlete train on an unstable surface is not wrong; it is just one element in a list of proprioceptive variables we can manipulate.

Uneven surfaces are just as stimulating as unstable surfaces. Having people work on different surfaces—ideally related to the terrain they will compete on—is a key component in altering proprioceptive input.

In addition to requiring input from the visual system, touch, and proprioceptive feedback, we need accurate information from the vestibular system.

Some of this comes from the eyes and is tied to the visual system, but data from how we are moving—particularly through rotation and in linear motion—is controlled by the utricle, saccule, and semicircular canals in each ear. The ability of this system to collect and transmit data can be compromised by an injury event, particularly when it involves trauma to the head.[199]

It is also effective to ask the athlete to change the head position during movement by looking up or down. Often, we might have an athlete perform single-leg balance activities while looking up, down, to the right, and to the left.

This change of head position will stimulate the semicircular canals of the vestibular system and challenge the neuromuscular proprioceptors contained in the ligaments and joints of the lower extremity.

Changing head positions mimics what athletes often do on the field—moving in one direction while looking in another.

Think of a wide receiver running down the field. His eyes are not closed and he is not standing on an unstable surface. He is running linearly, perhaps on an uneven surface, looking over his shoulder for the ball, running one direction while turning his head in another. Combine that with people running next to him or grabbing at him, plus the roar of the crowd, and you now have a significantly challenged the sensorimotor system.

We can apply these techniques to any athlete who is recovering from an injury and finding it hard to regain balance and proprioception.[200]

Vestibular rehab techniques are commonly used when rehabilitating concussion patients and are a highly specialized series of vestibular stimulation based on the specific trauma.

This type of vestibular rehabilitation is beyond the scope of this text, but it is important to be aware of the techniques. They can be used with anyone having trouble with balance and proprioception post injury.[201]

## DYNAMIC NEUROMUSCULAR STABILIZATION AND SOMATOSENSORY CONTROL

As we explored in Chapter Five, DNS enhances motion segment function and emphasizes the neurological aspects of stabilization in addition to the physical requirements. Using DNS techniques can also improve somatosensory control and the quality of movement outputs by recalibrating the inputs that are often disrupted by injury.

In his book *Therapeutic Exercise: From Theory to Practice*, Michael Higgins states that neuromuscular control—psychomotor, as we referred to it in the earlier chapter—does not just happen, but rather has a couple of precursors. One of these is:

> *"It requires somatosensory system input and works in conjunction with voluntary muscular activation to provide dynamic joint stability."*[202]

We cannot expect people to stabilize when not collecting accurate information about where they are in the environment, how the body is moving, and the tension the muscles are creating. Injury can disrupt all of these.

One of the ways DNS improves athletes' somatosensory control is by helping the body relearn primitive reflexes. The DNS school divides primitive reflexes into two subcategories: righting reflexes and postural reactions.

We do not only see righting reflexes in action with humans, but also in animals.

If you flip a dog over, it will immediately turn its head up and try to right its eyes. The same is true in children once they reach a certain developmental stage and can roll themselves over.

The human body is constantly trying to return to a homeostatic state. One way we do this is to get the head aligned so we can use our eyes to inform the brain about positioning and environment.

You can see an example of a postural reaction if you hold a baby upright, and then rotate the body face-forward as if falling. The baby will automatically extend the legs backward, shoot the arms forward and spread the fingers to prepare to break the fall. This is known as "the parachute reflex" and is a hallmark of "normal" development, usually occurring before a baby can walk. [203]

Primitive reflexes and reactions occur in infants and then either disappear, are integrated into more fundamental patterns, or continue throughout the lifespan.

The postural reflexes and righting reactions that disappear within the first year of life are integrated into more fundamental patterns, helping to support higher-level motor activities.

Although the actual reflexes are no longer present, the fundamental patterns they helped create are still available. By including activities that involve aspects of the reflexes, such as head movements during lower-extremity exercises, we can "tap into" the underlying reflexes to help strengthen motor control.

Next, the reflexes and reactions all have one thing in common: They are reflexive and do not require conscious thought to produce the motor response. These reactions were the low-level motor outputs—think spinal level motor control—that were created by the SMS to gradually progress from fundamental to transitional to functional postures as the body matures.

As higher-level motor responses were developed by the SMS, the reactions were integrated into these patterns. The reflexive nature of these primitive patterns can be put to use in our rehabilitation efforts if our interventions include activities that simulate the same type of reactions.

Choosing reactive techniques to help stimulate muscle activation and pattern engagement can be a very powerful technique for improving muscle activation and movement patterns. While we may not be working to actually restore primitive reflexes, any exercises that force the body to react to a stimulus will help facilitate our goals of muscle activation and improved movement patterns.

When an athlete is injured, such natural reflexes and reactions can cease to function well. Sending a patient to a DNS practitioner, or any practitioner who understands these concepts, can help restore the somatosensory and neuromuscular pathways by reinforcing these basic primal reflexes.

This advances the rehab by improving how the brain gathers and processes information about body positioning, balance, and stabilization in space.

There are other techniques such as Feldenkrais® and Neurokinetic Therapy™ that are similar and worth our consideration.

## YOGA—ORIGIN AND A MODERN APPLICATION FOR SOMATOSENSORY TRAINING

Yoga in its various forms can be helpful in improving a variety of movement dysfunction and has its place within the bridging-the-gap continuum.

Yoga is a poor choice if you want to work on power development or hypertrophy from a muscle-development standpoint. Yoga is fantastic for balance, proprioceptive training, organism and task constraints, and assisting in reestablishing the motion segment after injury.

I went to my first yoga class in 2002. We sat in a quiet room and held each posture for a long time. It felt like it was taking for-ev-er! I hated it and could not wait to get out of the room, promising myself never to return to yoga.

Five years later a studio opened near my house and a friend convinced me to go. I went kicking and screaming, going only because she bribed me with the promise of brunch and mimosas after the class.

That class was *nothing* like the earlier one. The teacher walked in sporting a handlebar mustache and a mullet, smelled of a certain herb, told us to come to the top of our mats, and turned on Snoop Dog. We proceeded to flow through one of the most difficult exercise classes of my life. I was dripping sweat by the end, proclaiming my newfound love of yoga.

I continued my practice intermittently, sometimes more consistently than others, until I obtained my 200-hour teacher certification in 2015. To this day, my favorite practice is Vinyasa flow. Mix that with a tattooed teacher playing good music and talking about how important it is to be a good to ourselves, others, and the earth…well, I am hooked.

Yoga arrived in the United States in the 1930s and was first studied as part of Eastern philosophy. It began as a movement for health and at the time promoted vegetarianism. In the 1960s, the countercultural youth movement became interested in anything and everything Eastern.

Within a few years, some of the more open-minded doctors began prescribing yoga for stress management. Since then, yoga hit the mainstream and became big business, with a yoga studio seemingly every few city blocks, and companies like Lululemon and prAna going global.

Yet, the struggle between Eastern and Western philosophies exists to this day. Western philosophies focus on anatomy and physiology and systems like musculoskeletal, neurological, psychological, and synthetic medications. Eastern philosophies draw from yin and yang, the five elements of fire, water, wood, earth, metal, and herbology—what many consider alternative medicine.

While Western medicine drills down to what is happening in a specific area with a microscopic view, Eastern medicine has a wider, more holistic macroscopic approach.

Despite their inherent differences, we can incorporate elements of Eastern and Western practices to help our athletes fully recover and improve long-term wellness. If you are new to Eastern disciplines, but are interested in incorporating them to improve somatosensory control, it is a great idea to start with yoga.

Yoga challenges the vestibular and proprioceptive systems by continually changing the participant's base of support and body position, and requiring a transition between postures while maintaining balance and motor control.[204]

One of the reasons yoga helps improve sensory input is that it forces the person to be mentally and physically present. One of the keys of yoga practice is to create an internal environment that minimizes external stimulation and distraction and encourages concentration and focus.[205]

> ## CLINICAL PEARL
>
> Why practice yoga?
>
> To get comfortable with being uncomfortable

## TYPES OF YOGA PRACTICES

There are many different types of yoga. If you are interested in testing yoga, try several different variations before declaring "I hate yoga" like I once did.

You may dislike one type of practice, but take to another.

The type I connect with most is *Vinyasa*, which centers on linking breath with movement. Every movement is connected with an inhale or an exhale. Inhalation and exhalation is used specifically to either deepen a posture or lengthen it. We use breath control in Vinyasa yoga to facilitate stability or mobility depending on the position.

*Yin yoga* is a slow-paced style that involves holding postures for five minutes or longer. Bernie Clark of *yinyoga.com* refers to the practice as being more yielding, passive, and quiet than other more active variations that emphasize the yang element.

It is believed to benefit the immune system, organ health, and, as with other types of yoga, stress management.[206] Yin yoga can be good for relaxation if you are feeling "tight," but remember, in our world of sports performance, things become tight for a reason.

Yin yoga can be calming and help us take much-needed time to slow down. If an athlete is sympathetic-dominant and finds it difficult to ease into parasympathetic recovery, yin yoga can help.

*Restorative yoga* involves active relaxation and often employs props or tools to support the body. This can be a nice option for people who have significantly limited range of motion and flexibility.

In the performance world, we are so afraid of static stretching that we have almost abandoned the technique.

We took several studies that showed an immediate or short-term decrease in power after static stretching, and as a result, we have literally tossed the entire technique out the window.

Static stretching, such as the kind used in restorative yoga, can be good if used at the right time and in the correct context. Immediately after performing the technique, static stretching appears to affect the visco-elasticity properties of the muscle and tendon unit.

However, when performed regularly and not before activity, there does not appear to be a change in visco-elastic properties, making static stretching a viable option on an off-day or after ballistic activity.[207]

Stretch-induced hypertrophy can occur, which can contribute to greater force production and increases in the velocity of muscular contraction. This was shown to apply across gender, age, and athletic level.[208]

Though static stretching should not take the place of soft-tissue work or be used before training or competition, it does have a place at the end of a non-competition or training day, or as part of the recovery phase of a periodization plan.

The static stretching employed in restorative yoga can also be useful when bridging the gap from rehabilitation to performance because it also emphasizes breath control, which can help improve the sensory input mechanism disrupted after injury.

We have touched on just a few yoga types; there are many more, including *Bikram, Ashtanga, Hatha, Iyengar,* and *Anusara.* Seek out, learn about and, most importantly, try several different types to see what fits practically and philosophically within your training and treatment philosophy.

## PRACTICAL APPLICATIONS OF YOGA IN THE BRIDGING-THE-GAP CONTINUUM

Now that we have looked into some different types, it is time to explore how you can apply yoga when working with athletes to enhance somatosensory control.

Before introducing yoga to your athletes, there are a few precautions. First, be aware of how each athlete's injury history might affect the ability to get into and sustain certain postures, and make this clear to the yoga practitioner. The last thing you want is to create a setback or to reinjure the affected area.

Second, be aware of your client's heat tolerance. If there is an underlying cardiovascular issue or problems like fainting or other signs of heat exhaustion or dehydration during hot preseason practices or games played in high temperatures, advise against styles of yoga in heated rooms that could further exacerbate dehydration.

Finally, as with every exercise you have your athletes perform in the gym, in the treatment room, or on the field, be sure that form comes above all. It is better for someone to spend weeks mastering a few basic postures than to rush ahead to more demanding positions and get reinjured. Remember, we are striving for greater body control, not less.

You do not have to become a yogi yourself, but please find a practitioner you trust so you can add yoga to your bridging-the-gap toolbox. For further reading on yoga, I refer you to Yoga Alliance at *www.yogaalliance.org*.

## SUMMARY

Overall, the somatosensory system is the driver to all movement. Sensory input dictates motor output.

The nervous system can select multiple ways to execute a movement pattern, allowing "healthier" systems more freedom of movement and therefore more functional variability that is vital to healthy movement.

There is no perfect way to perform a movement pattern. The nervous system will select an appropriate pattern based on the limitations of the organism, the task, and the environment.

Consider the qualities of touch, proprioception, vision, hearing, and vestibular when creating movement-program interventions.

# CHAPTER EIGHT
## OTHER CONSIDERATIONS FOR OPTIMAL FUNCTION

When Brian Grasso asked me to present at an International Youth Conditioning Association conference years ago, I asked him why he wanted me to speak since I do not work with kids. He said he knew I primarily worked with professional athletes, and that I must see problems I wish had been addressed when these athletes were younger.

He wanted me to talk about fixing issues that were once small and easily correctible—before they became big problems in the major leagues. Brilliant!

With this "start at the beginning" approach in mind, here are some must-do considerations for optimal function in athletes of any age and in any sport, whether pitching in Little League, college baseball, the minor leagues, or Major League Baseball. The takeaway is that we are never too young to start moving well, and it is rarely too late to start correcting fundamental positional and movement problems.

The elements in this chapter are things I do, assess, and address with every person I work with, despite gender, despite sport, and despite position. I am sure you could organize each of them somewhere along the *Bridging the Gap* continuum, but in my mind they form the foundation of my evaluation and treatment across the board.

The reason this section is here, at this point in the book, is that before I move on to further loading of a patient, I check on these fundamentals. If I try to load an athlete with weight or speed and these are not addressed, we see setbacks that cost us time as we move toward performance. These areas represent the beginning of my transition from rehab to performance.

In this chapter, we will break down the following topics:

*Breathing*

*Dealing with the diaphragm*

*Reeducating the diaphragm*

*Movement and breathing–Breathing and movement*

*Breathing and mobility*

*Breathing and stability*

*Paradoxical breathing and hip tension*

*Posture*

*Thoracic mobility*

*Lumbar spine rotation*

*The spine and shoulder mobility*

*The thoracic spine and the autonomic nervous system*

*Moving through the hips*

*Foot health*

*Education*

## BREATHING

When talking about universal considerations for all clients, we should start with the most elemental action of all: breathing. There is a reason Pilates and yoga place such a premium on breathing—if you can control your breath, you can control your life. This might sound a little "hippie," but it is a fact.

Emotions and actions can profoundly influence breathing. Think of when a person wakes up from a nightmare. The breathing will be fast and shallow, with the heart pounding in the chest.[209]

The same happens in sports. For example, in baseball, teams play 162 games in 183 days, not including spring training or playoffs. That is *a lot* of baseball. Then, finally, we move into October and a team makes the playoffs, where we hear the announcers say, "That guy has been here before." Having players on a team who have been under the pressures of a game of that magnitude can help the team stay focused, stay calm, and "play their game."

If a person on the team has never played in the playoffs, the intensity of a playoff game is higher. There are more people in the crowd than in the normal season—the game may be sold out. The athlete gets nervous because there is more at stake. The emotional aspect of what is on the line can change what is fundamentally the same thing the team has been doing since February—playing a baseball game.

When pressure is ramped up, the mind races, the heart rate goes up, and the breathing rate increases. It is difficult to control your racing mind, and you cannot consciously control your heart rate. What do you have to focus on? Your breath—you can slow down your breath.

Slowing your breath also slows your mind. Deep breathing stimulates the parasympathetic nervous system, which slows the heart rate. When you control your breath, you control your mind.

In isolated situations, rapid, shallow breathing is all right, and in the case of a fight-or-flight response to danger, it is necessary. We also see this breathing after a fast sprint. Increasing the respiratory rate is the body's first attempt at increasing oxygen levels in the system.

The trouble is, too many of us are stuck in this undesirable breathing pattern, where we are breathing faster than we should and more shallow than is ideal. We automatically breathe from the chest and neck, and take the diaphragm out of the equation, when it should be a prime mover in the breathing pattern.

The prime mover—in this case, the diaphragm—becomes a synergist, and the synergists to breathing—the scalenes, sternocleidomastoid, levator scapula, and more—become prime movers.

We have a psychomotor control issue that can eventually lead to neck pain and possibly back pain as well.

While athletes' resting respiration rates will vary slightly based on a number of factors, the range should typically be eight to 14 breaths per minute. Anything above this, the person is likely to be stuck in an apical breathing pattern—the type that involves the most movement in the upper chest and neck areas.

This apical breathing reduces the amount of oxygen in each breath, and the breathing rate becomes too rapid in an effort to make up for the lack of needed oxygen.

This also has consequences for soft tissue, the mental state, and the nervous system. The metabolic cost of apical or clavicular breathing is far higher than that of taking diaphragm-driven breaths, and that leaves us with less energy.[210]

There are also soft-tissue implications to apical breathing. The intercostals and other rib muscles can shorten, as can the pectorals and other chest muscles.[211]

As we have removed the job of the diaphragm as a prime mover and stabilizer and likely reduced activation of the abdominals, the body has to find stability elsewhere. For that, it will designate another prime mover—perhaps the hamstrings, the psoas, or the pelvic floor—to provide stability to the lumbopelvic hip complex.

Now we end up with excessive upper-quarter tension that manifests itself in chronically stiff traps, scalenes, levator scapulae, and other soft tissues of the upper and middle back and neck. Lower-back issues can also develop or are exacerbated.[212]

The cause of those nasty headaches your clients are struggling with? For that, you can often look to the tension created by the apical breathing.

This so-called "stress breathing" tells the brain that we are in a continual state of high alert. The sympathetic state becomes far more dominant than its parasympathetic "rest and digest" counterbalance, making it difficult to relax and recover.

This in turn affects heart rate and elevates levels of stress hormones such as cortisol. We feel anxious and panicked because our faulty breathing mechanics are *telling* us to feel that way.[213]

Many athletes live in a sympathetic state. There is constant stimulation at home, on the field, from the press, and from self-imposed expectations. The athletic body is under constant stress from the rigors of training and performing.

Sleep is often compromised due to travel and odd schedules. Under-recovery or over training, or both, is common. Breathing—yogic breathing, specifically—has been shown to balance the autonomic nervous system by influencing heart rate, altering CNS excitation, and altering neuroendocrine functions.[214]

This is why breath control is an important therapeutic exercise: It can solve or reduce the impact of all kinds of issues that other therapies cannot touch.

It has the potential to reset the nervous system, enhance mood and energy levels, reduce anxiety, lower blood pressure, improve immune system function, improve rib, thoracic spine, and neck mobility, and much more.[215]

This all starts with the diaphragm.

## DEALING WITH THE DIAPHRAGM

It might sound weird, but I *love* the diaphragm. The lats used to be my favorite muscle until I discovered how complex and extensive the role of the diaphragm is in everyday function.

For starters, it is anatomically freakish, running from the underside of the ribs to the T6 vertebrae, then down to L2 on the left and L3 on the right.

As an anatomy refresher, the psoas runs all the way from the front of the femur up to L1, which means there is a direct anatomical connection between it and the diaphragm. When I say that breathing, lumbar stability, and the hip are connected, you can take it literally.

As you know, when a body lacks primary stability, it will create it. The diaphragm is not only meant to be a respirator, but is also a stabilizer of the spine. However, a body will always choose breath over stability, and if it has to give up stability from the diaphragm in favor of breath, another part of the body has to replace it.

What does the diaphragm attach to? The psoas. How many of our clients say they have "tight hip flexors"? Most of them, and of course they do! They are trying to create secondary stability in an environment that inherently lacks it.

Then we try to "massage and stretch the psoas" and wonder why nothing changes. If we do make a change, we wonder why it is short lived.

If we do not address the improper use of the diaphragm, we will never decrease the hip flexor tone we spend so much time trying in vain to alter.[216]

We are not only dealing with downstream tension in the hip flexors on the anterior side, but also stiffness in the lower back and inefficient position of the glutes on the posterior side. When combined with the excess tension at the front of the hips, this fundamentally alters the lumbopelvic-hip relationship and can lead to a cascade of other biomechanical issues farther up or down the kinetic chain.

Then, because of the diaphragm's attachment in the thoracic spine, it is also tied to the musculature of the middle back—not to mention its link to the ribs, intercostals, and upper abdominals on the anterior side. If we are not taking deep breaths, the ribcage does not expand as it is supposed to; the ribs become stiff and the thoracic spine becomes hypomobile.

The same is true on the reverse side of the body in the soft tissue of the thoracic spine. If a client is struggling with tightness or soreness in the middle back, the breathing pattern is likely the culprit or at least a contributing factor. Such a mobility restriction can limit thoracic extension, flexion, or rotation, or produce the feeling of being "stuck" in thoracic extension or flexion.

This is a big problem in many sports, particularly those like baseball and tennis or any kind of paddling.

## REEDUCATING THE DIAPHRAGM

We first need to reeducate the diaphragm to function as both a respirator—the prime mover for breathing in and out—and a stabilizer. Ideally, the diaphragm should set the tone for the entire lumbar-pelvic complex, but when we are stuck in apical breathing, this is not the case.

Obayashi et al[217] looked at 26 swimmers and measured their spinal curvature and isometric trunk strength before and after inhalation and exhalation respiratory training using a spirometer. A spirometer is a device used to train both inhalation and exhalation muscles via resistance during breathing activities.

They performed this training three times per week for 10-minute sessions, for four weeks. They found that the participants in the exercise group had a decrease in thoracic kyphosis of 5.5 degrees, and a decrease in their lumbar lordosis by 3.3 degrees. By stimulating the local core stabilizers and retraining the diaphragm through resisted activity, they could significantly change posture.

While this is a small study and needs to be taken in the context of healthy subjects, it is nonetheless an interesting one. It needs to be replicated with more simple spirometers for training purposes, and needs to be recreated in subjects with pain. However, it begins to give us some insight that breath-based training has the potential to have significant implications for both structure and function.

## MOVEMENT AND BREATHING, BREATHING, AND MOVEMENT

*Breath facilitates movement.*

*Movement facilitates breath.*

*Breath facilitates stability.*

*Stability facilitates mobility.*

### Breath Facilitates Movement

Breathing should be three-dimensional. When trying to emphasize diaphragmatic breathing, it is common to ask an athlete to lie down on the floor and breathe so the belly rises and falls, but this is not the only place there should be movement. Yes, we call it "diaphragmatic breathing," but it is also costal. There should be some lateral, anterior, and posterior expansion in the chest cavity as well. Our lungs do not live in our abs.

If you put a tape measure around a person's ribcage and ask for a maximal inhale followed by a maximal exhale, you should see a change in expansion by 2.5 centimeters from one extreme to the other.[218]

If you do not see this change, you can assume one of two things: Either there is a true, possibly structural hypomobility of the rib cage, or there is a dysfunctional movement pattern preventing proper use of the diaphragm as a prime mover for respiration.

When thinking about the relationship between breathing and movement, remember, this is a two-way street. If you want to see how breathing can facilitate movement, sit on the edge of a chair with great posture and take in a big breath. Your chest will rise toward the ceiling and you will get thoracic extension.

If you forcefully exhale, your chest drops and you get a little spinal flexion. If you think about breathing into your left side, you will feel yourself perform a slight sidebending to the right. If you put your hand on your ribs on the right side and focus on breathing into your hand, you will feel yourself slightly bend to the left. Breath clearly facilitates movement.

With this breathing-and-movement relationship in mind, we can use inhalation to achieve better thoracic extension while mobilizing a kyphotic client.

We might also use it to enhance thoracic rotation left and right. In addition, we can use exhalation to improve thoracic flexion.

## Movement Facilitates Breath

On the flip side, movement can also facilitate breathing. If you again sit on your chair, bend to the left and breathe, it will be your right side that feels like it is filling with air.

If you slump over, you will notice your breath is directed toward the posterior side. Now if you sit up straight in the chair with your chest sticking out, you will see your anterior chest expanding as you breathe in.

In essence, movement or position can influence breath.

Think about a person who has a flat thoracic spine, which is reduced thoracic kyphosis. Consider what branch of the autonomic nervous system lives in the thoracic spine: the sympathetic nervous system—our flight or fight system. When a person is in a position of constant thoracic extension, this is pushing the sympathetic nervous system toward the "on" state.

Encouraging a more flexed thoracic position can decrease this constant stimulus to the sympathetic nervous system and can help reduce the stress and anxiety—see later in this chapter for more on the relationship between the thoracic spine and the autonomic nervous system.

It can also allow people to break the shallow, apical breathing pattern in which they may be stuck. If you put people into a slumped position like a child's pose, they are forced to breathe into the posterior thorax.

This will help mobilize the thoracic complex and encourage some parasympathetic activation via deep breathing.

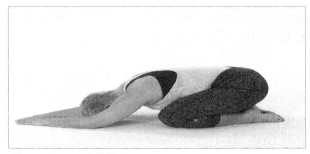

**Photo 8.1—Child's Pose**

*Child's pose is one of the first poses taught in a yoga class.*

*Despite being a position of rest, it may not feel restful to many people.*

*Child's pose requires significant ankle, knee, hip, and spine mobility, and it may prove to be a very challenging position for your athletes. You can use folded blankets or towels as support behind the knee or hips when needed, working your way toward the full expression of the pose as they gain more mobility.*

You will notice that people might get anxious because they cannot figure out how to breathe in this position—you have taken their compensatory movement pattern away from them.

If this happens, flip the child's pose into side lying and have them hug their knees. This will make them a bit less claustrophobic, yet still give you some of the results you are looking for when using postural-directed breath for improving thoracic flexion.

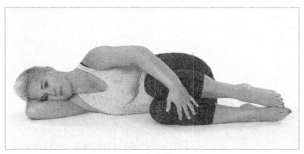

**Photo 8.2—Side Lying Child's Pose**

*Performing child's pose in a side lying position can be less demanding on the joints than the full pose. In addition to being easier on the ankles, knees, hips and spine, it is an easier position in which to breathe.*

*When in child's pose, people may have a difficult time breathing if they lack proper thoracic spine and rib mobility.*

*This can create anxiety and result in the opposite effect you were intending.*

*Performing the pose in side lying allows more room to breathe, improves rib and thoracic spine mobility, and is a nice regression to the full pose.*

This is just one example of how various movements and postures can help adopt and facilitate better breathing.[219]

In essence, movement or positions can profoundly affect breath.

## Breath Facilitates Stability

Facilitating stability is an additional way in which diaphragmatic breathing can improve performance. If you put your hands on your obliques, which have two subsets—internal and external—and then powerfully exhale, you will feel those muscles contract. This forceful exhalation gets into what is called the "expiratory reserve volume."

That may be a term you have not heard, so let us review some fundamental breathing nomenclature.

As you sit and read, you are respirating. Unless you are really excited about this book, you should not be taking overly deep breaths while reading. This normal breathing pattern for exhalation and inhalation is called tidal volume.

Tidal volume involves a concentric contraction of the inhalation muscles, where the diaphragm and external intercostals are prime movers, followed by an eccentric contraction during the exhale.

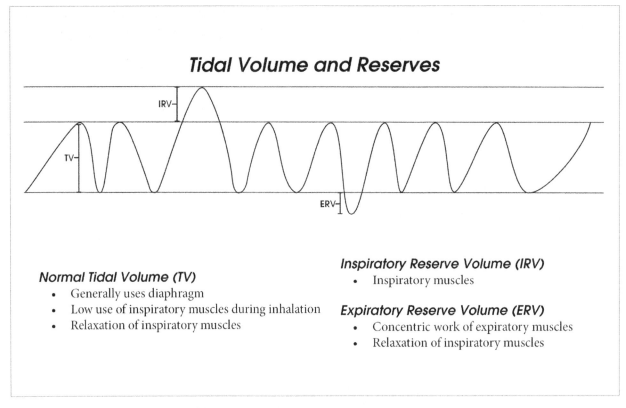

**Figure 8.1—Fundamental Breathing**

*Understanding common terminology about breathing is necessary for proper communication and understanding of the breathing process. The above graph is a simple representation of common terms and muscle action as it relates to normal breathing, forced inhalation, and forced exhalation.*

If you take a deep breath, you are getting into the inspiratory reserve volume. The lungs can hold way more air than what we naturally take in per breath. Tapping into the inspiratory reserve volume requires a concentric contraction of the inhalation muscles with the diaphragm and external intercostals as prime movers and sternocleidomastoid, scalenes, and pec minor as accessory muscles. This is followed by an eccentric contraction of the inhalation muscles.

It is not until we utilize this expiratory reserve volume that we actually get a concentric contraction of the expiratory muscles—the internal intercostals, abdominals, and quadratus lumborum.

When exhaling all the air you are holding, you will feel a contraction of the abdominals, forcefully expelling the excess air from the lungs.

We can use this expiratory reserve volume to contract the abdominals, get the thoracolumbar junction in a neutral position, and work on core stability by having the person maintain this position while normally inhaling and exhaling. The body's innate need to inhale due to pressure changes in the lungs will cause us to automatically inhale when needed.

After getting into this "neutral" position, we can begin to get the "body diaphragms" in parallel.

**Figure 8.2—The Four Diaphragms**

*If we look at the concept of a diaphragm being a sling, we see multiple slings in the body. The arch of the foot creates a diaphragm-like support on the bottom of the foot.*

*The pelvic floor creates a sling supporting the underside of our torso.*

*When we dissect the underside of the neck and jaw, we see there are multiple muscles that look much like the pelvic floor, supporting the neck, head, and mouth in a similar fashion.*

*These "diaphragms" should be in parallel to obtain optimal static posture. When the "diaphragms" are no longer parallel, such as with forward head, excessively lordotic spine, anteriorly tilted pelvis, and flat feet, the body is not starting from a neutral position.*

*Movement then compensates to make up for the less-than-ideal starting position.*

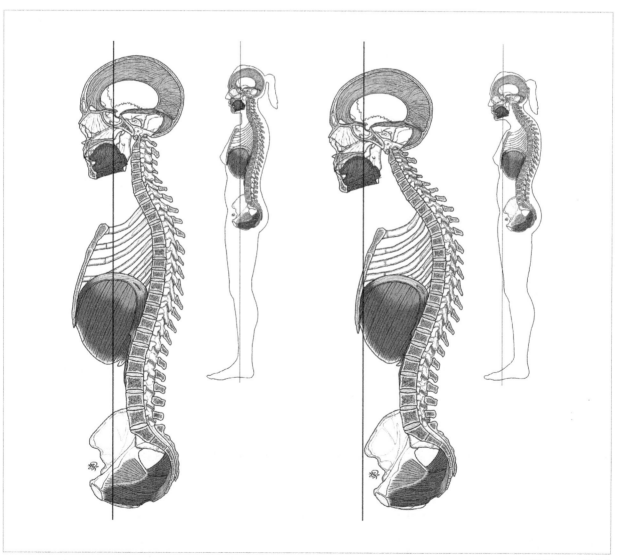

© Danny Quirk

This may be a new idea for you. Think about the arch of your foot, the pelvic floor, the actual diaphragm, the roof of your mouth, and top of the tongue.

When these are all parallel with each other, we are in a neutral spine position. When these things are not parallel, we get into trouble with both stability and mobility.[220]

> ## CLINICAL PEARL
>
> The "four diaphragms" should be in parallel. If they become out of parallel, a "neutral" posture has been lost.
>
> - Arch of the foot
> - Pelvic floor
> - Respiratory diaphragm
> - Tongue and roof of the mouth

This concept of having multiple diaphragms in the body has been a key to my teaching the idea a neutral spine to my patients.

Think of the torso as a canister. The top of that canister is the actual diaphragm. The bottom of that canister is the pelvic floor. If these are not in parallel with each other, we will have torso stability issues simply due to posture and positioning.

If the head juts forward and the tongue is not in parallel with the pelvic floor and diaphragm, the person may have neck issues or thoracic pain. If the arch

of the foot is overly pronated, overly supinated, or rotated out due to hip or knee positions, there will eventually be lower-extremity pathology and pain.

Keeping the "diaphragms of the body" in parallel is an essential concept in body neutrality.

## Stability Facilitates Mobility

As we have discussed, mobility and stability go hand in hand. It is difficult to create powerful, efficient movement on an unstable surface, and it is difficult to create mobility without stability in the system. As Gray Cook teaches us, stability issues are often disguised as mobility problems, and vice versa.

## PARADOXICAL BREATHING AND HIP TENSION

Sometimes I see a client whose issue is not just breathing apically, but the brain and body have reversed the normal mechanical rise and fall of the diaphragm when breathing.

In people dealing with a paradoxical breathing pattern, the belly button moves in during inhalation, causing a hollowing of the stomach and the chest to stick out. Then on the exhale, the belly moves outward again. This decreases the inherent stability within the lumbar spine and thoracolumbar junction, restricts airflow, and leads to greater stability and movement or mobility issues in the entire system.

The diaphragm should move and function from the central tendon. When

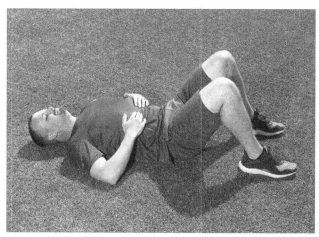 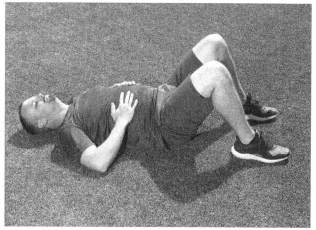

**Photo 8.3—Paradoxical Breathing Patterns**

*Normal inhalation is associated with a natural expansion of the abdomen as the diaphragm descends and pushes on the abdominal contents. On exhalation, the diaphragm rises, releasing pressure in the abdominal cavity, allowing a "moving in" of the stomach.*

*Paradoxical breathing is the opposite of this natural mechanism; upon inhalation, the stomach goes in, pushing against a diaphragm. This prevents the diaphragm from descending, so the only option to get air into the lungs comes from using accessory muscles in the neck and chest to expand the rib cage.*

*These synergistic muscles of breathing now become the prime movers, creating a less-than-optimal breathing strategy that can result in fatigue, poor trunk stability, back pain, and neck tension.*

breathing optimally, the attachments of the diaphragm should remain stiff while the central tendon moves up and down. The attachments of the diaphragm are the ribs—this does not mean "fixed," as the ribs should move.

However, the ribs should remain more fixed relative to the central tendon. If the opposite occurs and the central tendon remains fixed, the ribs flare and there is excessive movement at the thoracolumbar (TL) junction.

Every time a person takes in a breath, the back extends at the TL junction, causing decreased stability at the torso. The body diaphragms are no longer in line.

As the ribs flare forward, the back extends, the pelvis can become anteriorly tilted, and excessive movement is fostered at the TL junction.

The cycle continues to perpetuate itself; paradoxical breathing causes ribs to flare and excessive motion at the TL junction. The excessive movement at the TL junction decreases the inherent core stability of the system.

The psoas or hamstrings increase tone to provide stability because the body is more focused on respiration than stabilization. Eventually muscles get stiff and we discover a structural issue that all started from a paradoxical breathing pattern.

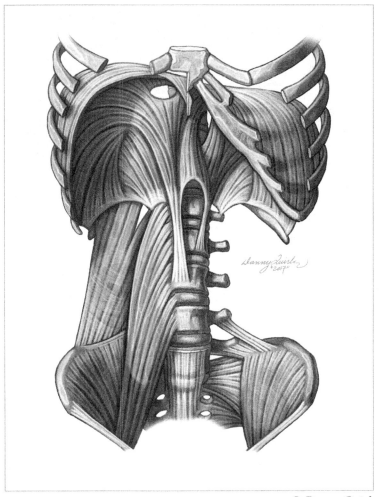

*© Danny Quirk*

**Figure 8.3—Diaphragm and Posture**

*The diaphragm is a muscle that can be trained like any other muscle in the body. It has multiple functions, given its intense attachments to both visceral and somatic structures.*

*Breathing issues can result in decreased pulmonary function and fatigue, as well as musculoskeletal postural issues and pain. There is some evidence that breath training can actually alter the position of the spine.*

To decrease the hip stiffness involving the psoas and hamstrings that the system has created due to lack of stiffness in the trunk, we need to first stop the paradoxical breathing.

Once we give the trunk the proper breathing mechanism, everything else usually falls into place. The hip musculature will relax, as there is now enough stiffness in the system proximal to the hips. They are now free to move as they are supposed to, acting as prime movers or synergists of the hip.

We can fix a paradoxical breathing pattern by giving the client verbal and tactile cues to reinforce the correct sequencing involved in normal diaphragmatic costal breathing.

Because of the direct connections from the diaphragm to the psoas, working on one will affect the other. Improving hip mobility and hip function can decrease the synergistic actions of the trunk, allowing a more natural function of the diaphragm and hip.

Exercise options used to promote this include:

- *Spinal neutral breathing with use of expiratory reserve volume*

- *Single-leg hip lift*

- *Cook hip lift*

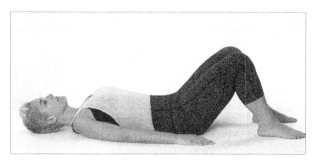

**Photo 8.4—Spinal Neutral**

*Ask the athlete to anterior and posteriorly tilt the pelvis. Find the excursion of movement and have the person stop somewhere between the two extremes of motion. In this position, look for your client to breathe normally. Tactile cues on the stomach and rib cage may be used to get the natural "push out" of the abs on inhalation, and "inward movement" on exhalation. Nothing is forced, allowing the breath to become natural.*

*Once that occurs, you can have the patient exhale maximally, which will engage the oblique muscles. This is known as expiratory reserve volume—forcing more air out of the lungs than what is naturally exhaled.*

*By activating the obliques on this forced exhale, the patient can feel the position of the spine and maintain this position moving forward.*

*The key at this point is to breathe naturally while being able to maintain this "spinal neutral."*

*Once spinal neutral is established with a natural breathing pattern, the organism can be challenged accordingly. This can occur by changing the position of the legs or arms.*

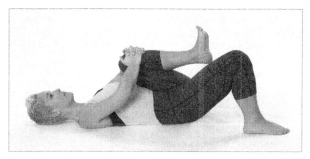

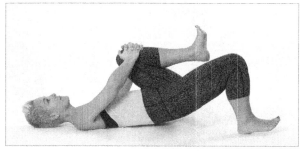

**Photos 8.5a and 8.5b—Cook Hip Lift**

*Once a body can tolerate different positions in supine, we can challenge the system even more. By adding in a more complex hip mobility exercise as pictured, we can begin to work on hip mobility with trunk stability at the same time.*

## POSTURE

English physiologist Sir Charles Sherrington said it best[221] in 1906:

*"Posture follows movement like a shadow."*

The concept of good posture is not new, but it has fallen out of favor in recent years. In this day of functional movement and movement efficiency, people care less about static posture—other than your grandmother, who likely still "tuts" at you to remind you to sit up straight.

However, what we have lost sight of in this movement-focused climate is the question of how can we have an efficient movement pattern after starting from an inefficient position.

In short, we cannot.

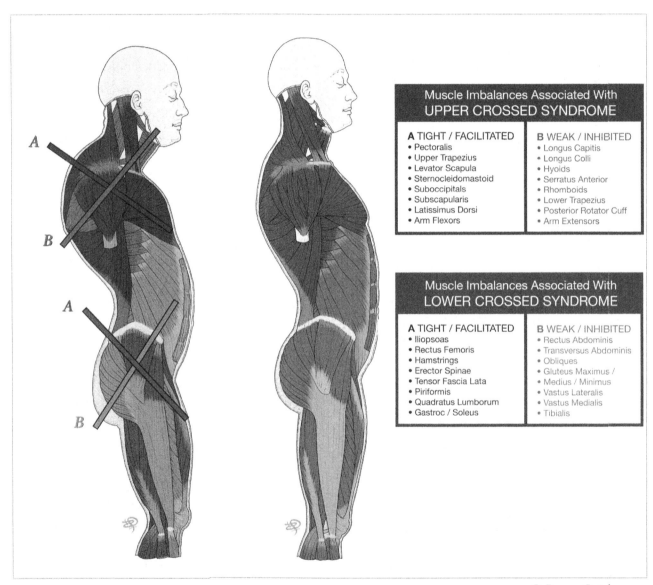

© Danny Quirk

**Figure 8.4—Upper and Lower-Crossed Syndromes**

*Upper- and Lower-Crossed Syndromes were described by Vladimir Janda in the early 1980s. This concept represents the body's natural tendency to get "tight" and "weak" based on postural faults.*

*While these concepts are not dogmatic, meaning there are other compensations that can be seen, they are often observed clinically and can be a great starting point for a professional to observe postural deviations.*

Vladimir Janda developed his concepts of Upper- and Lower-Crossed Syndromes in 1987, described earlier on page 69, and the concepts continue to hold true.

Although we can argue *why* muscles become tight and weak—everything is driven by the nervous system—we continue to see these patterns clinically and therefore they are worth discussing. Proper static posture is the starting foundation for proper dynamic movement. The two go hand in hand.

The book *Assessment and Treatment of Muscle Imbalances: The Janda Approach* (2010) is an excellent resource for all of Janda's teachings, including the concept of the crossed syndromes.

In his idea of the Upper-Crossed Syndrome, the suboccipitals, upper trapezius, and levator scapulae, along with the pec major and minor, become tight, while the deep neck flexors, lower trapezius, and rhomboids become weak.

Stiffness is introduced into both the anterior and posterior chains. This is a naturally occurring syndrome when people have what is considered "poor posture." A forward head position, elevated and protracted or winging scapula, increased cervical lordosis, and an increase in thoracic kyphosis are common compensations seen in people with this syndrome.

Upper-Crossed Syndrome can lead to cervicogenic headaches, shoulder impingement, neck and upper back pain, as well as joint dysfunction, specifically at the atlanto-occipital joint, C4-C5 segment, cervicothoracic junction, glenohumeral joint, and T4-T5 segment.

Janda noted that these areas of stress in the cervical and thoracic spine correlate with anatomical changes in the vertebrae as they transition from one area to the next—a good example of structure affecting function.

Lower-Crossed Syndrome is recognized by tight thoracolumbar paraspinals and hip flexors, accompanied by weak abdominals and glutes.

Anterior pelvic tilt, increased lumbar lordosis, and knee hyperextension are often associated with Lower-Crossed Syndrome. The L4-L5-S1 junction, sacroiliac joints, and hip joints are often dysfunctional. Low back pain and pelvic or sacroiliac pain are other common symptoms.

Pavel Kolar was a student of Professor Janda's, as well as of Karl Lewit and Vaclav Vojta, and is the creator of DNS, described on page 104. Kolar describes "good" posture as a co-activation of everything: a co-activation of the flexors and extensors, a co-activation of the abductor and adductors, and a co-activation of the external and internal rotators.

Good posture is different for everyone, depending on anatomical structure. When antagonists are in balance, the system is happy.[222]

Karl Lewit taught us the idea of the "old" versus "new" systems.[223] The "old" system consists of the flexors, the adductors, and the internal rotators.

When a baby is born, it is positioned in a little ball, with all of the "old" musculature system in a tonic phase. It is not until a baby hears its mother's voice or sees something shiny when it is on its belly that it begins to push itself up, and turns its head in search of the new sound or sight.

This activates the "new" system—the extensors, abductors, and external rotators. These systems balance at around three months of age. Everything we do when we are in pain, fearful, tired, or after a neurological compromise like a stroke or cerebral palsy brings us back to the "old" system.

Think about when you hurt your arm: You probably cradle it in front of you. When you are tired, you slump forward in your chair. When you are fearful, you cower. Pain, emotion, and neurology are all driven toward this "old" system.

This is why we focus so many of our interventions on the "new" system.

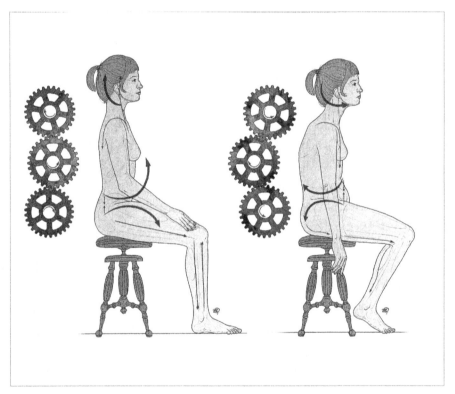

© Danny Quirk

**Figure 8.5—Brügger's Cogwheel**

*Brügger's Cogwheel is a great depiction showing how one part of the system can affect the positioning of another. We can often focus on nonpainful areas of the body to address more painful ones if needed. Pain can lead to protective posturing, eventually causing structural changes.*

*Also, poor posture itself can lead to nociceptive chains or trigger points in the body that are neurologically driven painful areas. It goes both ways. We can massage these painful areas and potentially get results, or we can change the neurological input into the system, change static posture, and therefore decrease pain throughout the body.*

Many of our therapeutic interventions activate or support extension, abduction, and external rotation patterns. Much of the "new system" muscles are those that tend to get weak in the crossed syndromes as defined by Professor Janda. The "old system" muscles tend to get tight.

Alois Brügger, a Swiss neurologist, used the idea of a cogwheel to describe the inter-dependability of the spine on itself. He encouraged patients to adjust the lower cogwheel—the pelvis—into a clockwise position, allowing the chest and head to follow into good posture.[224]

Brügger evaluated posture and movement on a neurophysiological basis, rather than on specific pathology. He taught that the neurophysiological overload caused pain and thus a protective posture and positioning due to this pain.

Therapeutic exercises can address these overactive and tight hypertonic or underactive and weak hypotonic issues that present themselves despite the accompanying pathology.

The upper-extremity Brügger exercise shown in Photos 8.6a–8.6d is a favorite for combating Upper-Crossed Syndrome, posterior-chain weakness, or anterior-chain over-activity or tightness. The band is wrapped around the hands so there is no gripping of the band.

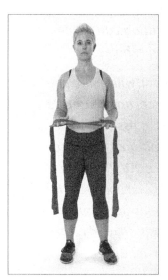 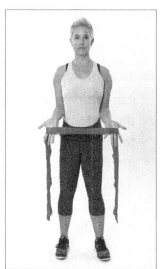 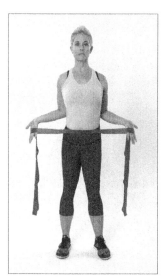 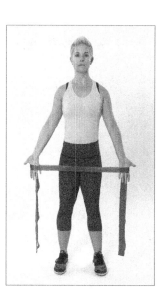

**Photos 8.6a–8.6d—Brügger's Upper-Extremity Exercise**

*In the upper-extremity Brügger exercise, we use the concept of muscle irradiation to train the entire posterior chain versus strengthening one muscle. By activating the entire neurological chain, we can decrease the "tight" painful areas on the anterior side.*

*These concepts continue to repeat themselves, over decades, across the world and in orthopedics and neurological-based patient populations: activate muscles that are weak versus stretching and massaging those that are tight.*

*Things become tight and painful when the antagonist of those areas become weak. If we address these areas as a whole, we can impact the neurological considerations of the body, which drive the musculoskeletal system.*

We are trying facilitate the extensor mechanism, or the "new" system, and we do not want one part of the system stimulating the flexor mechanism, or "old" system.

The exercise is performed in stages. First, the palms are supinated, fingers and wrists extended, shoulders externally rotated, and elbows extended. Then, the order is reversed very slowly, emphasizing the eccentric portion of the exercise with elbows bent, shoulders internally rotated, fingers and wrist returning to neutral, and palms pronated.

Other exercises you can use to promote better posture include:

- *Floor slides, then progress to...*

- *Wall slides*

- *Wall walks*

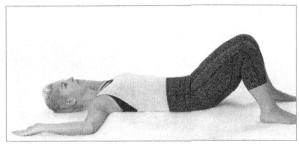

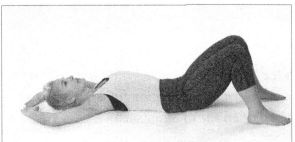

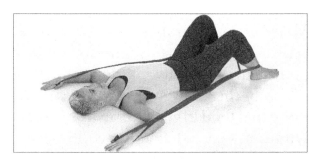

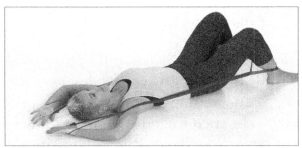

**Photos 8.7a–8.7d—Floor Slide**

*Allow the patient to lay supine, with knees bent and arms overhead in a 90/90 position as shown. The first step is to make sure the person can obtain the 90/90 position at the shoulder. If not, active external rotation can be performed while the person exhales.*

*This exhale on movement will utilize the expiratory reserve volume, and therefore the abdominal muscles to assist in maintaining core stability and good thoracolumbar positioning. Once 90/90 shoulder movement is achieved, on exhale, the person can slide the hands up above the head into a diamond position, and return to the 90/90 position on inhale.*

*This can be repeated as necessary to activate the posterior chain while improving anterior chain mobility. Once the person is able to perform this exercise properly with full mobility and good thoracolumbar positioning, you can extend the legs, which will challenge the thoracolumbar positioning even more.*

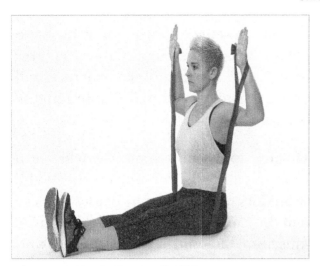 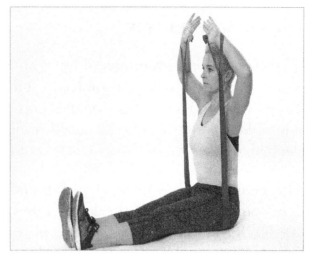

**Photos 8.8a–8.8b—Wall Slide**

*The wall slide is a progression of the floor slide. Once the person is able to perform the exercise properly in supine with knees straight, move to a position against the wall, with the upper extremity in the same position as was used in supine. Knees are bent.*

*The same inhalation and exhalation is performed with the corresponding movement as described above, adding gravity to the system, which increases the difficulty of the exercise. Once this exercise is mastered, have the person straighten the legs in sitting, which will significantly challenge the system.*

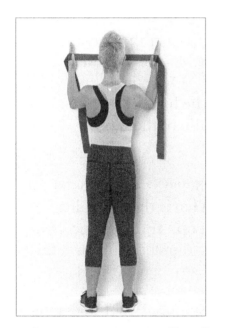 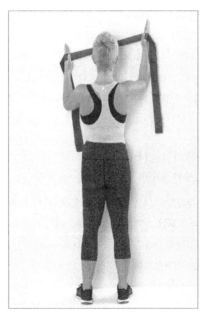 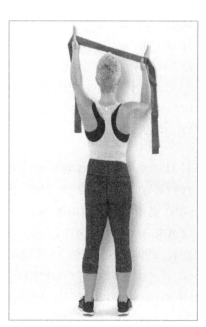

**Photos 8.9a–8.9c—Wall Walk**

*In the wall walk, the person will have an elastic band wrapped around the wrist, not gripping the open end of a band. Ask your client to place the ulnar side of the forearm on the wall, with hands at about shoulder height.*

*Using expiratory reserve volume to assist in thoracolumbar positioning, the person "walks" the arms up the wall until the elbow gets to about the height of the eyes, and then walks back down the wall. This exercise can be repeated to fatigue.*

## THORACIC MOBILITY

In today's world dominated by computers, smart phones, and tablets, even those of us who are active spend a considerable amount of time hunched over electronic devices.

The head falls forward and the shoulders round; we cut off the lower lobes of the lungs, emphasizing an apical breathing pattern with a shallow chest or neck that decreases the ability to use the entire lung capacity and move through the full excursion of the ribs. As a result, the ribs get somewhat "bound down" and no longer perform the needed movement required for full inhalation and exhalation.

The ribs attach to the thoracic spine via the costovertebral joints and the costotransverse joints. Two connections per rib to the thoracic vertabrae, multiplied by 24—12 ribs on each side—means 48 connections from the ribs to the thoracic vertebrae.

If the ribs are not moving well, the thoracic spine is not moving well either, and if a large number of these connections are compromised, there can be a massive decrease in rotational capacity of the thoracic spine, placing additional stress on the shoulder complex and lumbar spine.

This also works in reverse, in that a hypomobile thoracic spine will limit rib mobility. Once this happens, the body has to figure some things out. We will always find a way to breathe, as this is essential to keeping us alive.

In the absence of any other way, a default apical breathing pattern emerges because the immobile structure will no longer allow optimal diaphragmatic breathing.

During apical breathing, we will see a superior and inferior movement of the shoulders and shoulder blades. There will be an over-activity of synergistic muscles, including the scalenes and sternocleidomastoid, as the body tries to increase the respiratory rate to get enough oxygen to take care of normal body processes.

When we decrease the depth of breath, the rate has to increase in order to make up for it, with a greater energy cost to the musculoskeletal system.

This over-activity of the scalenes pulls the first rib up toward the clavicle and can decrease the space where the brachial plexus lives. Over time, numbness and tingling in the hands can occur due to the compromise of these neurovascular structures.

Think about being at your computer for even an hour. What is the first thing you do when you get up? You probably bend backward, push your chest forward, take in a breath, and stretch your neck.

When we are stationary for too long, our joints do not move the synovial fluid around as much as needed for nourishment of the joints, and the muscles get stiff from being in one position.

When we do this long enough or repetitively, that tightness turns to rigidity.

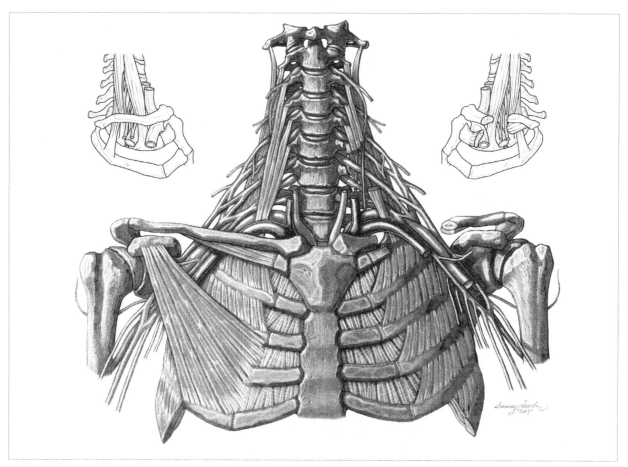

© Danny Quirk

**Figure 8.6—Thoracic Outlet**

*The term "thoracic outlet syndrome" is actually a misnomer.[225] The thoracic outlet is the inferior thoracic aperature, at the bottom of the ribs where the diaphragm is connected. The thoracic inlet is defined by the boarders of the first ribs, T1 and the manubrium, and is also known as the superior thoracic aperature.*

*However, clinically, pain as a result of compression of the neurovascular structures in this area is known as thoracic outlet syndrome (TOS).*

An actual change in the mobility of the thoracic spine will occur and eventually the spinal structure can change, causing a permanent rounding of the spine.

We cannot spend our lives looking at the floor, can we? The body is a master compensator and will figure out how to get the eyes level with the horizon. Our eyes need to look forward, and therefore we will extend the neck, shortening the suboccipital region, and placing tension in the upper traps.

In addition, the paraspinals get overactive and we become hypermobile at the thoracolumbar junction. The paraspinals get so much use, they become hypertrophied. The result is what look like "sausage paraspinals."

155

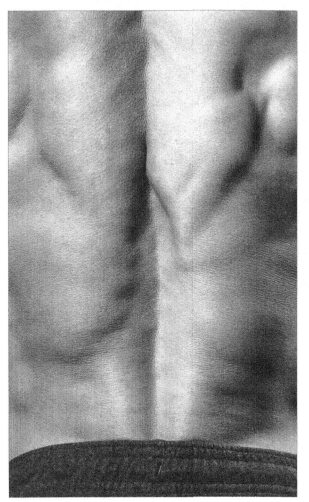

**Photo 8.10—Hypertonus of the Paraspinals**

*Gross movement is often favored over fine movements in the body. When the body does not have the ability to control the individual fine motor skill of refined movement, large gross movements often substitute.*

*In the absence of control of spinal intrinsic activity, large paraspinals take over to create gross movement.*

*Overuse results in hypertrophy, hence the large "sausage paraspinals" often seen in our clients.*

*These hypertrophied paraspinals are an indication of poor fine motor control of the spine.*

## LUMBAR SPINE ROTATION

There are about two degrees of rotation at each segment of the lumbar spine, with the exception of approximately three to five degrees at L5–S1. This gives us a prospective total of 10–12 degrees of rotation, assuming tissue function is normal.

The facet joints of the lumbar spine are in the sagittal plane. This sets them up to allow flexion and extension, but not rotation or sidebending. Simply put, the lumbar spine is not made for rotation.

Look at the vertebrae in Figure 8.7.

One of the reasons we get excessive motion and hypermobility at the lumbar spine is due to loss of motion at the thoracic spine and hips. Because this area of the back is not supposed to handle such a rotational load, we now see back pain, stenosis, herniated discs, and degenerative conditions start to emerge.

The tension continues downstream to the glutes and hamstrings and starts to alter the lumbar-pelvic relationship. This can then begin to compromise function at other joints below the lumbar area, such as the hip, knee, and ankle.

Now consider the general osteokinematics of the thoracic spine—the movement of the bones in the thoracic spine. Based on the orientation of the facet joints, this area is set up well for lateral sidebending.

That is not to say sagittal- or transverse-plane motion does not occur at the thoracic spine. It just means it is not the

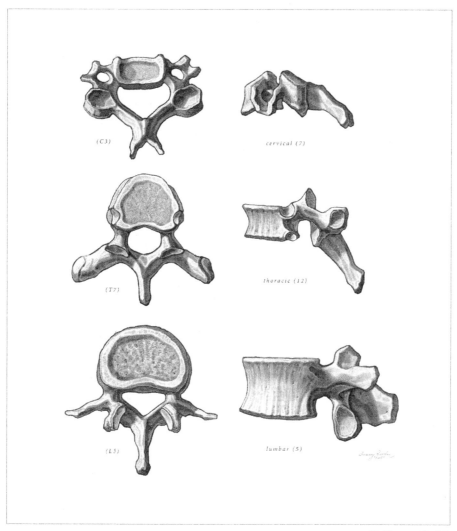

*© Danny Quirk*

**Figure 8.7—Vertebrae**

*The top sketch is a typical lower cervical vertebra. Note the small vertebral body and facet joints in the transverse plane. The cervical spine is not created for weight bearing, and is well designed for rotation as whole.*

*As we move into the thoracic spine, the vertebral body gets slightly bigger to support more weight of the body and movement in the upper extremity. The facet joints begin to move toward the frontal plane, making the thoracic spine great for side bending.*

*By the time we get down to the lumbar spine, we have a large vertebral body that supports the weight of the torso and leg movement, as well as facet orientation now moving to the sagittal plane. This structure functionally sets up the lumbar spine for flexion and extension.*

main movement based on the anatomy of the facet joints.

From a rotational standpoint, there are about two degrees of movement at each segment of the thoracic spine. Since there are 12 thoracic vertebrae, that gives us up to 24 degrees of potential rotation at the thoracic spine.

This is a generalized assumption, as ribs get in the way and alter this math.

If the thoracic spine becomes hypomobile, the body will make up for this limitation by forcing more motion elsewhere, typically at the lumbar spine or at the C5–C6 junction in the neck.

Finally, the cervical spine is beautifully set up for rotation. Those facets are generally in the transverse plane, and the anatomical setup of C1–C2 is designed for rotation.

While the lumbar spine is anatomically set up for sagittal-plane motion, the thoracic spine is set up for frontal-plane motion, and the cervical spine is set up for transverse-plane motion, we have an unbelievable structure for three-dimensional, total-spine movement.

That is, it works if everything is working correctly. When one part of the system is not functioning well, another part needs to pick up the slack…and here come the problems.

## THE SPINE AND SHOULDER MOBILITY

When evaluating and treating the upper quarter, we must think about the associated osteokinematics of the joints.

As you sit in your chair right now, perform the following movements to feel these concepts. First, sit up tall, as you were probably a bit flexed after sitting. In order to achieve full, unimpinged bilateral shoulder flexion, we must have

thoracic extension; so, reach overhead with your right arm and pay attention to the extension and rotation involved.

To achieve full unilateral shoulder flexion, we need both thoracic extension and ipsilateral rotation. In the case of right shoulder flexion, we need thoracic extension and right thoracic rotation. To get unilateral shoulder extension and internal rotation, we need thoracic flexion and contralateral rotation…left rotation—reach behind your back with your right hand to feel this.

Now, perform the same movements when slouching in a position of thoracic flexion. You do not get that same full motion, do you? You might feel a pinch in your shoulder, or even pain there. Your spine is stiff in this position and does not move well.

In essence, we need thoracic mobility for shoulder mobility.

Associated osteokinematics come into play when gaining range of motion. If in treatment we only focus on the single joint associated with the pain, we may be missing a large part of the picture.

For example, consider the shoulder mobility test of the FMS, where you compare the client's backward reach on each side. If someone performs poorly on this test, yet when lying down you find 90 degrees of shoulder external rotation and 45 degrees of internal rotation, the limiting range-of-motion factor is most likely not the glenohumeral joint. It is probably the thoracic spine.

If your interventions continue to aim at the glenohumeral joint, your client may get somewhat better, but maybe not 100 percent. Merely prescribing a set of shoulder exercises or pulling the joint this way and that might provide temporary relief, but it is doing little to uncover the root of the problem or to restore full range of motion.

In fact, continued efforts directed at the glenohumeral joint could actually cause a *hyper*mobility, further exacerbating the problem.

I have recently changed my approach to thoracic spine mobility. I previously used a peanut-shaped tennis ball tool, recommending that people self-mobilize

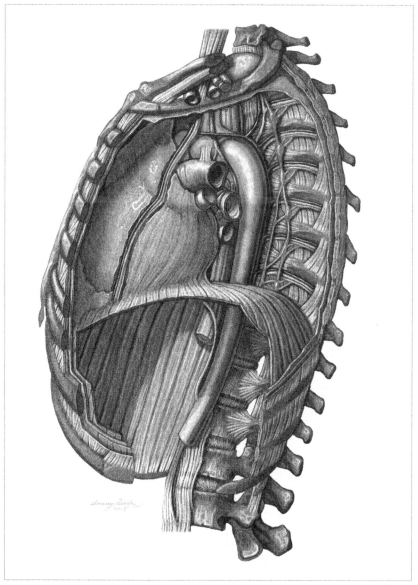

*© Danny Quirk*

**Figure 8.8—Mediastinum**

*The posterior mediastinum is a space created by the diaphragm on the bottom, the peri-cardium on the anterior side, the T5-T12 vertebrae posteriorly, the pleura laterally, and an imaginary line from the sternal angle to T4.*

the thoracic spine, as well as prescribing a lot of thoracic foam rolling. I still use these tools, but with caution, and not with every athlete. Read on to find out why…and what to do instead.

## THE THORACIC SPINE AND THE AUTONOMIC NERVOUS SYSTEM

The posterior mediastinum is a space that contains some interesting structures, specifically the sympathetic trunk.

The sympathetic system is anatomically dominant in the thoracolumbar area, while the parasympathetic system is anatomically dominant in the craniosacral area.

People who have flat thoracic spines or a decrease in thoracic kyphosis have a decreased posterior mediastinum space. That does not leave much room for the sympathetic trunk and ganglia, and they are likely being constantly stimulated.

This keeps our athletes and patients in a state of "emergency." The last thing these people need is more stimulation of the sympathetic nervous system.

With such athletes, we actually need to restore thoracic flexion. We can do this with the expiratory reserve volume, exhaling as much air from the lungs as possible, and focusing on segmental spinal flexion.

If we need to improve mobility in these clients' thoracic spines, we should focus more on rotation exercises, such as those below, rather than forcing them into more extension, since they are already stuck in extension.

With the client who is overly kyphotic, it is tempting to mobilize into more extension as well. The problem with this is if a person is already in a sympathetic state, we may be unnecessarily stimulating the sympathetic nervous system by pushing into more extension with either manual therapy or peanut-like devices.

I am not saying I do not use these anymore; I do. I am simply more selective on whom I use these treatments, and quite often go to breathing or rotational exercises to restore thoracic and rib mobility, rather than jamming the person into extension, decreasing the space of the posterior mediastinum, and placing an already sympathetic athlete into a more sympathetic state.

Some exercises to promote thoracic mobility include:

- *Prayer rotation*
- *Upward facing dog*
- *Downward facing dog*
- *Seated flexion balloon blowing*
- *Standing serratus squat*

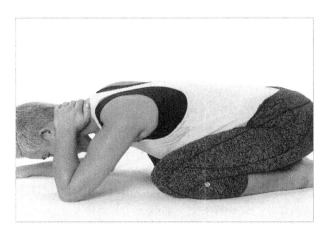

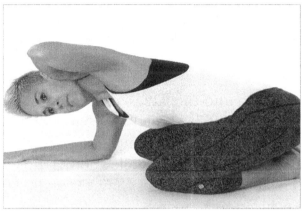

**Photos 8.11a–8.11b—Prayer Rotation**

*Place the client in a modified child's pose position. Maximal knee flexion, hip flexion and lumbar flexion should be attainable; however, you can use props as needed to achieve this end-range position.*

*Place the hand of one arm near the face, so the shoulder is relaxed down at the side. The other hand should be placed behind the neck or head. The client rotates toward the ceiling, looking under the axilla, following the movement with the eyes.*

*Movement is focused at the thoracic spine, and inhalation or exhalation can be used to enhance the movement. The client returns to the starting position and repeats to both sides as needed.*

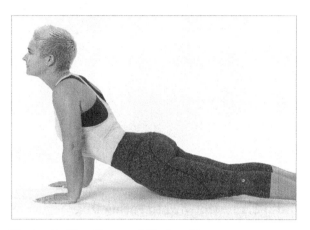

**Photo 8.12—Upward Facing Dog**

*Upward dog is a classic yoga pose and is often combined in sequence with downward dog. Start the movement in Chatturunga, which is a low plank position. Have the client push the chest through the hands toward the wall in front, looking up toward the ceiling. Hands push into the ground, giving significant depression to the shoulder girdle.*

*The thoracic spine is extended and the eyes look up to the ceiling. The motion can be accompanied by an inhalation to enhance the movement. The weight should be on the top of the feet, with the thighs lifted in the air. Be mindful that your client does not "dump" into the lumbar spine, creating excessive pressure and ultimately pain in the low back.*

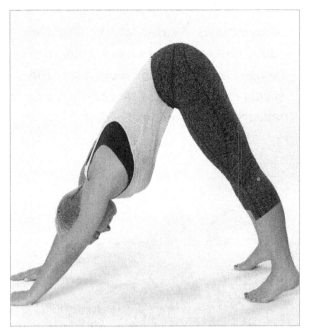

**Photo 8.13—Downward Facing Dog**

*Typically done from an upward facing dog position, the client pushes through the hands so the hips move to the ceiling and the person is in an upside-down pike position. The chest pushes through the arms, placing the shoulders in an end-range position of flexion and with maximal thoracic extension.*

*Tension is placed throughout the entire lower posterior chain, with the client feeling a stretch in the hamstrings and calves as well. This position can also be achieved from a high plank position, where the client simply pushes back into the position described and then moves forward into a high plank to move out of the pose.*

Ultimately, the spine—specifically the cervico-thoracic junction and the thoracic spine—and shoulders move hand in hand. The shoulders cannot express their full range of mobility for a wide variety of activities of daily living if the spine is not stable and mobile enough to let those upper extremity movements happen.

## MOVING THROUGH THE HIPS

Before you even started reading, you must have known we would discuss the squat pattern. The squat has been so thoroughly discussed, dissected, and debated, and yet correctly performing it is still elusive for our average clients.

My first trip to Asia was in 2011 when I went to Beijing to work with the Chinese Olympic Committee. What is the first thing you do once you get through customs after a long flight? You go to the bathroom.

I walked into the ladies' room and went to the first stall, opened the door and saw a big hole in the ground. Interesting. I went to the second stall, another hole. Third stall...a hole. Fourth stall, a beloved toilet. Score!

It was the same story everywhere I went that was not a major tourist hub. In all the Olympic training venues and outside restaurants, there were several stalls with holes in the ground and, if I was lucky, one with a toilet.

During my two weeks at the Olympic training center in China, I saw some extreme orthopedic pathologies and movement dysfunctions. Nevertheless, no matter how "messed up" an athlete was, I would typically see a beautiful squat pattern. Of course the Chinese have a beautiful squat pattern! They have to use it all the time in order to use the toilet.[226]

Excretion of waste is a fundamental human need and is as important as breathing. Those of you who have watched an elderly family member or a sick friend lose this basic function know it is devastating and humiliating.

We are about to get down and dirty here as we talk about defecating. I promise you this will come full circle—stay with me.

The body will typically figure out how to defecate even if the process is not efficient. Trying to use the toilet standing up would be very difficult. We naturally get into a squat pattern to assist the process, creating intra-abdominal pressure and assisting with peristalsis of the digestive tract, which allows us to eliminate the waste that was not absorbed during the digestive process.

Western culture created a device to assist this process: the toilet. This ubiquitous device brings the ground up to us so we do not have to squat all the way to the floor, yet in the process, this has compromised our ability to squat.

Many cultures simply use a hole in the ground and because they do, they maintain the ability to squat throughout a lifespan. In addition, many of these societies also squat while they eat, which further maintains the mobility of the hips that we in Western cultures consistently strive for, yet find so difficult to achieve and sustain.[227]

There was an ayurvedic lecture at a yoga conference in Phoenix recently—ayurveda is an ancient practice of holistic medicine that takes into account the mind, body, and spirit when dealing with health and wellness.

At one point in the lecture, the instructor said, "We are a constipated society."

That is so true. So many people in Western cultures have difficulty eliminating waste for many reasons, including consuming too much processed food, not having enough fiber, and not getting into the proper position to eliminate waste from the body.

Continuing with the thought that squatting assists in defecation, if we squat deeper, we should be able to boost the elimination process.[228] If we improve elimination, we get rid of more waste. If we get rid of more waste, we decrease the bloating, gas, and other digestive issues typically present in many people in the Western society.

How many of your clients are lactose intolerant, have acid reflux, or are sensitive to gluten? There is a reason we do not find a gluten-free or dairy-free menu when in Korea or China, and, in a roundabout way, one of the reasons has to do with the squat assisting the process of elimination. Of course, gluten and dairy are not huge components of their diet anyway.

What do we do in Western society? We create a toilet so we do not have to squat down to eliminate waste and then realize perhaps that was not the best idea after all, so let us create *another* device to get us back in the proper squat position—the Squatty Potty!

Go to the website *squattypotty.com* to take a look. It is a fantastic invention that takes us back to our squatting roots, promoting the digestive health we need to help with a myriad of visceral and musculoskeletal issues.

However, even though I appreciate the concept, we should remember that other cultures have no need of a secondary device such as a Squatty Potty.

Hip mobility is vital for lumbar spine health. If we do not have the proper hip mobility to perform necessary functions like defecating, we will get the mobility elsewhere because this bodily function is not optional. We externally rotate our hips, round our lumbar spine, and compensate our way through life.

I am not saying the lumbar spine should not flex—of course it should. Based on the anatomical setup of the lumbar facet joints, the lumbar spine is beautifully organized for flexion and extension. However, the spine will have to do flex, because the hips or thoracic spine cannot move.

The hips are set up beautifully for rotation, and the hips are where we drive our power production from, as we will flesh out in the Fundamental Advancement chapter beginning on page 191.

If the hips and thoracic spine cannot rotate, that movement is sent to the lumbar spine, and that usually does not work out very well, especially for the L5 S1 segment. We end up with hypermobility in the lumbar region and eventually the resultant disc and facet degeneration.

Hip and thoracic mobility are vital to the health of the lumbar spine.

## FOOT HEALTH

Foot health is another imperative to address in our clients. We know from Vladimir Janda's work that there is a high concentration of proprioceptors at the suboccipitals, the sacroiliac joint, and the feet.[229] We accumulate information into our afferent nervous system from our feet being in almost constant contact with the ground.

Our afferent system, which involves sensory information, will have a direct impact on our efferent system, which is motor output, meaning sensory input dictates motor output. If our sensory input is diminished or incorrect, our motor output will be inefficient and incorrect. Our athletes' feet must have our attention during the path from rehab to performance.

In 2011, there was a surge in barefoot training, in large part due to the extraordinary success of Chris McDougall's excellent book, *Born to Run*. Everyone was wearing Vibram Five Fingers or other zero-drop shoes, not only during training, but also when walking around the mall, on their way to work, and whenever they would have ordinarily been wearing a traditional shoe.

When diving into the research with my colleagues at EXOS, you can only imagine our delight when we found this amazing article from *American Journal of Orthopedic Surgery* dating back to 1905 entitled *Conclusions Drawn From a Comparative Study of the Feet of Barefooted and Shoe-Wearing Peoples.*[230]

The article shows that wearing minimalist shoes or barefoot walking is not a new concept in the performance world. For over a hundred years, people have known that wearing shoes, although great for many reasons, also has its pitfalls. The pictures in the article comparing the feet of people who had never worn shoes with those who did showed astonishing structural differences.

The long axis of the great toe should bisect the heel. The toes should be the fattest part of the foot. Our arches should not be dragging on the ground.

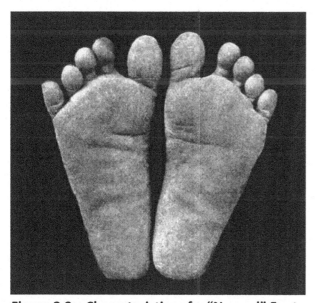

**Figure 8.9—Characteristics of a "Normal" Foot**

*Although shoes are a fantastic creation to protect our feet from the elements, they have also created unnatural pressures, altering the structure and therefore the function of the only part of the human body that touches the ground.*

*Notice from this 1905 image of a Negrito adult, the widest part of the foot should be at the toes, with toe separation, skin folds at the arch, and with the long axis of the big toe bisecting the heel.*

*In the modern world, our feet often do not look like this, with their flattened arches, big toes pointing off to the side, and smaller toes unable to abduct.*

Clearly, that is not the case once we began wearing shoes.

Wait: Shoes are not all bad. They protect our feet from the elements of the external world. However, our culture went from always being barefoot to always wearing shoes, most of which have elevated heels. We have profoundly altered our foot structure and function with this change in footwear.

For natural foot movement, we should wear shoes with wider toe boxes that allow for a natural splay and that have flat soles that do not elevate the heel. If an athlete is accustomed to a higher heel stack when training, you can gradually reduce to heel-to-toe drop in the footwear until the drop reaches a minimal number, such as two to four millimeters or even zero-drop shoes.

However, this adaptation will take time, and few of us can go back to never wearing shoes. To make a successful transition to a minimalist or barefoot program, we first need to prepare our feet, lower legs, hips, and lower back.

This is where a foot-care program comes into play. Like any movement pattern, posture, or external device, nothing is inherently wrong with our shoes. Similar to when we cannot get out of a movement pattern or cannot transition well from one to another, over time, things can become problematic.

It is not that people should never wear shoes. I have a hot pair of Christian Louboutins that I will never give up. However, I cannot use them every day and when I wear them, I need to do some foot love the next day.

Once of the strategies I use is the short foot drill. The concept of the "short foot" was introduced by Vladimir Janda and is an important idea to teach to your clients and athletes.

Creating a short foot allows us to use all of the intrinsic muscles in the foot, taking stress and overuse away from the long foot muscles, such as the extensor digitorum or flexor digitorum. The short foot concept allows the small muscles of the foot to support the natural arches, which can also improve balance.[231]

Restoring the proper position of the first metatarsal is also important.[232] This is especially vital for athletes who wear cleats and women who cram their feet into pointy-toed shoes.

Compressing the toes will lead to pointing the first ray in a more medial position, often creating a bunion. When we have a bunion, we do not properly transfer force from the rear foot to the forefoot; we "fall through" the midfoot, further driving the compensation.

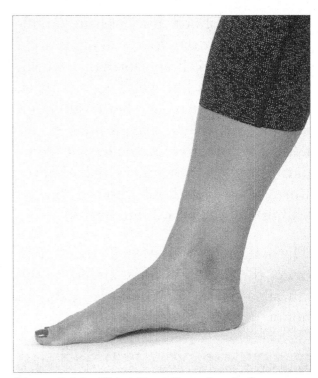

**Photo 8.14—Short Foot Exercise, Before**

*Note the flat position of the foot and the internally rotated position of the distal tibia.*

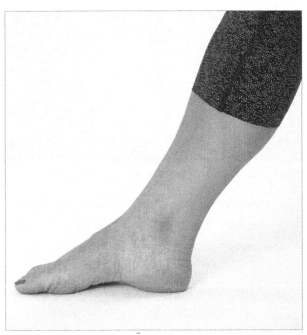

**Photo 8.15—Short Foot Exercise, After**

*The client is asked to make a "short foot" by pulling the heel closer to the toes.*

*This movement will make a "cave" under the arch of the foot, creating skin folds in the arch. The distal tibia externally rotates, which is sometimes an easier cue for people to visualize. The toes should remain relaxed, being able to move without gripping the ground while performing the short foot exercise. If the toes grip the ground, the person is using the long toe flexors to create an arch, rather than the short foot intrinsics we are trying to activate.*

Repositioning of the first ray is imperative in restoring proper foot function.[233] One of the best techniques I have found to do this is using Yoga Toes®.

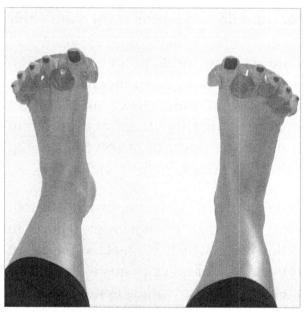

**Photo 8.16—Yoga Toes**

*Yoga Toes or similar devices can help stretch the toes into abduction, specifically allowing the first ray to be positioned in a neutral position.*

*Sitting with these toe spacers at least once daily, starting at about five minutes*

*in duration and working to 30 minutes, can stretch cramped feet that are normally in shoes all day.*

*Once we restore this range of motion, the short muscles of the foot have room to do their job, allowing activation and strengthening of these important proprioceptive muscles.*

You will not find many specific products mentioned in this book; however, when I find one that works like no other, I talk about it. I give Yoga Toes to just about any athlete who has foot-and-ankle dysfunction, such as the inability to perform a short foot, or who has a poorly positioned first ray. My patients wear them for up to 30 minutes per day and we watch the changes unfold.

I have seen a huge improvement in many athletes' ability to control the foot's intrinsic muscles and manage foot pain after using these toe stretchers, which is why I continually recommend them to my clients.

Once attaining the first ray in neutral, improving the first metatarsophalangeal joint extension is our next goal. The best way to do this is with archetypal postures, which Phillip Beach describes beautifully in his book *Muscles and Meridians.*[234]

Although when you first begin with these, they certainly do not feel like resting postures, static resting postures several times per day, will, over time, make huge changes to mobility, stability, and overall function.

## CLINICAL PEARL

If you activate the glute med, the foot intrinsics will fire and create a "short foot," or a foot with a supported longitudinal arch. Glute med activation and foot function go hand in hand.

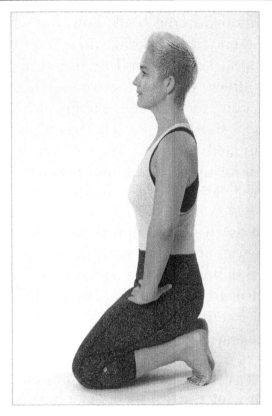

**Photo 8.17—Toe Sitting Posture**

*Toe sitting requires maximal toe extension with full stretch of the plantar fascia. Full ankle dorsiflexion, knee flexion, and hip flexion are also required. These end ranges of motion are often painful to people because they have lost full range of motion in these joints.*

I regularly use the Toe Sitting Posture shown in Photo 8.17 as a static positioning activity.

In this position, people are on their knees, toes curled under so they are in maximal first metatarsophalangeal dorsiflexion, maximal ankle dorsiflexion, full knee flexion, and full hip flexion.

They are sitting upright, which requires lumbar stability and an element of thoracic mobility into at least a neutral position so they do not fall forward. This is not a resting position at all! Many of your athletes will not be able to get into this position due to hip, knee, ankle, or foot issues.

Our joints lose mobility over time; we get a functional joint immobilization from not fully using the entire motion that should be present at the joint, stiffness sets in, as does joint degeneration. Pain ensues, usually limiting motion even more. This is an awful cycle that could be prevented if we simply never lost the ability to obtain and maintain some of the postures of rest that Phillip Beach describes.

Finally, massage is important in foot care. Whether or not you believe in reflexology, which is massage based on the concept of reflex points in the hands and feet, there are many benefits of massaging and mobilizing the bottom of the foot.

Sticking with purely biomechanical and fascial reasons, the tissue on the bottom of the foot needs to be pliable to maintain a functioning Windlass mechanism.

JH Hicks first described the Windlass foot mechanics in 1954; it is an integral part of normal foot function, allowing proper weight transfer throughout the foot. Maintaining suppleness of the tissue is an important part of this function.[235]

The following are exercises and tools that help eliminate the stiffness in the soft tissues of the foot and activate much-needed foot intrinsics.

Using a hard ball with no give for the soft-tissue component can cause bruising, pain, and other issues, so start with a softer, "grippy" ball that provides the desired stimulus—something like Jill Miller's Yoga Tune Up Therapy Ball. You can help your client can build up tolerance from there.

- *Short foot, shown earlier in Photos 8.14 and 8.15*

- *Toe spreading*

- *Other toe movements–first metatarsophalangeal joint extension, fourth-toe flexion and vice versa (not shown)*

- *Ball rolling*

- *Cowboy posture*

- *Kneeling posture*

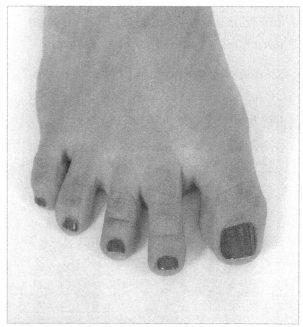

**Photo 8.18—Toe Spreading**

*Having the ability to abduct the toes is a crucial yet often lost skill. By abducting the toes, we are activating the small foot intrinsic muscles of the foot that help support the arches for proper force absorption and production.*

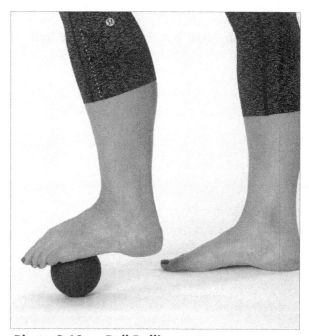

**Photo 8.19a—Ball Rolling**

*Adding rolling on a ball to your foot health repertoire can reap multiple benefits. Improving the mobility of a stiff foot will help with force absorption during all activities, including walking.*

*Stimulating the bottom of the foot stimulates the L5S1 nerves, and potentially can help with low back pain.*

*Increasing the pain pressure threshold will also decrease local foot pain.*

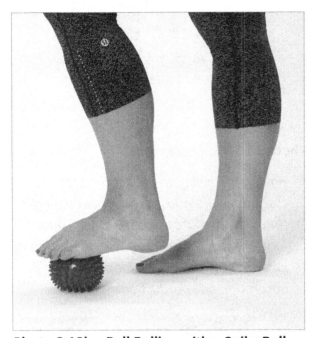

**Photo 8.19b—Ball Rolling with a Spiky Ball**

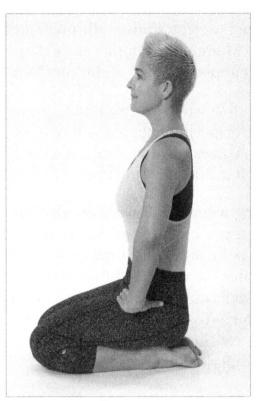

**Photo 8.20—Kneeling Posture**

*Kneeling posture is similar to toe sitting with the exception of the toe position. In this posture, the toes are not curled under—the person is sitting on the top of the feet, with the ankles in full plantar flexion instead of in ankle dorsiflexion.*

*This posture can be supported by placing pillows under the knees to alleviate discomfort due to end-range knee flexion and then progressed into the full pose.*

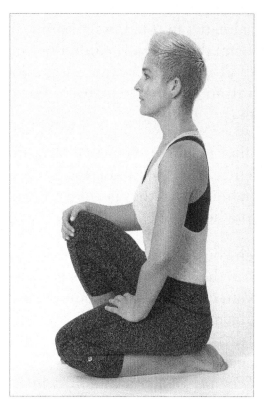

**Photo 8.21—Cowboy Posture**

*Cowboy posture is a combination of kneeling posture on one leg, with the opposite leg in full flexion as pictured. This posture should be stable and comfortable and was historically used to perform work in front of the body.*

## EDUCATION

Nelson Mandela said, "Education is the most powerful weapon we can use to change the world." I cannot think of a more true statement.

Pain is scary; when people are in pain and lose movement function, they are fearful—afraid they will never be out of pain, never recover full motion capacity or get out of the current state. They

catastrophize, thinking of the worst possible scenario they can conjure. In turn, this can increase pain perception.[236] Education takes much of that fear away because it gives the unknown a name.

After we define an issue, we can establish a plan so the client can work toward a goal. On the path from rehab to performance, we must educate our clients about the probable diagnosis and the roadmap we have created for them.

Once people understand a plan, they can buy in and can become active participants in their destiny. They gain control not only of the process, but also of the likely outcome.

Often athletes discuss a past surgery and have no idea what was done or how it may have impacted the condition. They are unsure of what structures were "fixed" or what it did to move them further toward the return to performance.

In my practice, almost daily I pull out an anatomy text or app to show people why they are feeling what they are feeling. This clarifies something that has taken on a life of its own in their heads, and helps make it tangible. Once they can associate what they feel with what I describe, a light bulb flicks on. I hear things like, "No wonder that hurts. I might need to stop doing it."

Education also gives people a better idea of what they *can* do. When people are empowered with knowledge and can actively participate in their movement-based homework, they can work on addressing their issues for the 23 hours a day they are away from the clinic or gym.

This removes the expectation that *we* will fix them, and reminds them they have the power to heal themselves. That is one of the greatest gifts we could ever give to our clients.

## SUMMARY

These are the considerations I think about with every client, no matter where we are between rehab and performance. Posture, breathing, the thoracic spine, hip mobility, foot care, and education are at the foundation of my clinical and performance practices.

Addressing these issues with clients who are already in pain will significantly influence their overall health. Preventing issues in these areas would stop a lot of pain from ensuing in many of our performance clients.

Monitoring these elements early in an athletic career could also prevent issues down the road as they get older and have less physical ability to adapt to change.

When you are unsure what to do, going back to these fundamental basics should put your client on a good course to health and balance of the system. We should address these areas prior to moving onto the performance-based aspect of the *Bridging the Gap* continuum, which we will cover next.

# CHAPTER NINE
## FUNDAMENTAL PERFORMANCE

As we have discussed, the first thing we need to do with people in pain is to get them out of pain. Next, by addressing the motion segment, we make sure they acknowledge and use the injured body part with the rest of the system.

During this process, we verify that the correct muscle is firing at the right time—this is *psychomotor control.* We take into account the nervous system and how it is processing sensory information—this is *somatosensory control.* And, we consider all things physically, mentally, and socially that could be playing a factor in this process—this is *the biopsychosocial aspect.*

We know the body will alter its motor output in the presence of pain. Therefore, it is almost impossible to work on motor skills or strength when someone is in pain. However, it is mandatory to work on localized strength in the area of injury once we control the painful experience.

Please refer to Chapter Four, page 65, for an overview of localized strength testing and muscle performance as outlined by Florence Kendall. Fundamental strength of local musculature is the base for any type of foundational performance or total-body strength expression. One cannot be strong as a whole if the individual parts are weak.

Once we have reestablished the strength of the motion segment, it is time to turn our attention to rebuilding fundamental performance capacity. As kettlebell pioneer Pavel Tsatsouline suggests, we need to target strength first.

When people are strong enough to perform the activities required in a sport, we can then layer on universal athletic competencies like acceleration and deceleration and sport-specific skills.

In this chapter, we focus on building strength and power as a whole, so our athletes are prepared to translate strength and power into athletic movement. We will also discuss how we apply the concept of periodization to create and implement a structured, goal-oriented recovery timeline.

## COMING TO GRIPS WITH SUPERCOMPENSATION

When it comes to sports performance or everyday activities like loading boxes for a move to a new house, each muscle must have the basic, foundational ability to carry out the task we are asking it to do.

Do the muscles we need to recruit have the ability to sufficiently fire against gravity with resistance?

During standardized manual muscle testing, can each muscle perform at a foundational "five out of five"[237] strength? If not, we need to do some basic strength training. We cannot begin to address speed or power without first having basic strength.

If your client is not ready for resistance training, it will be difficult to build strength—or in the case of injury rehabilitation, to rebuild strength.

During the bridging-the-gap process, be aware that the injured body part might not be ready for resistance training, but there are usually other areas that are able to handle strength work. Your programming should focus on maximum maintenance or strength gain in areas that are not injured, while protecting injured tissue where necessary. This is why the bridging-the-gap model is not a continuum, but more of a checklist of items to address prior to returning an athlete to sport.

To see strength gains, we need to understand and employ the basic concept of supercompensation. This is a process that first requires the introduction of a training stress, and then we look for the body's reaction to and recovery from that load. At its core, supercompensation simply means adaptation to a progressive training load.

After we apply a stress during training, there is an immediate physiological decline in performance.

**Figure 9.1— The Slide**

*The Slide is the graphic representation of this book. It shows the different phases of return to play after an athlete is injured.*

*This is not a true continuum—people do not have to "pass" one stage to move onto the next. Several sections can and should be developed at the same time. However, they all must be addressed to have a comprehensive plan for return to play.*

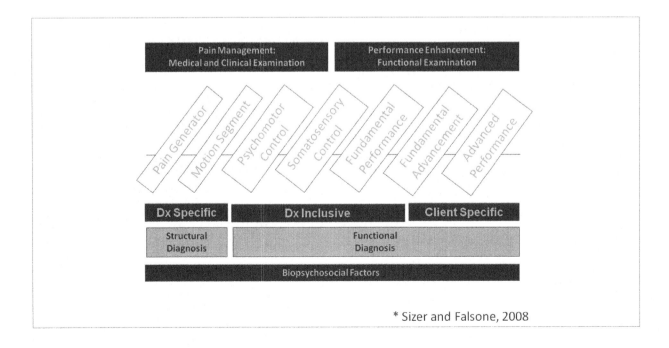

* Sizer and Falsone, 2008

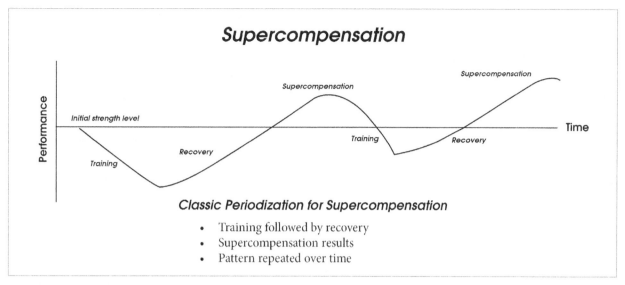

**Figure 9.2—Supercompensation**

*Supercompensation is what every athlete is striving for within a training model. We need to stress the system in order to see changes. However, we cannot continually stress the system without giving the body times to rest, recover, and adapt to the applied stimulus.*

*This positive adaptation to stress is coined "supercompensation," and can be achieved with a detailed, well thought-out performance plan.*

This is followed by a recovery period.

The body then adapts and performs with more efficiency and greater power output in following workouts or competition. This is due to an improved ability to manage stress, as well as the physiological changes the body made when recovering from the previous stimuli.

If well timed, we delivery the next training stressor when the body can continue to build on the previous one, making the tissues bigger, faster, or stronger. If the next stimulus is introduced too early, the body will not be able to recover and the athlete may become over trained—or, truly, under-recovered—thereby causing a negative physiological effect.

## PRIORITIZING PLANNED RECOVERY

Planned recovery is an important concept to discuss with your athletes, and even more so when returning from an injury. An athlete's psychological mindset is always to "do more."

When players get hurt and have to watch from the bench while teammates practice and play, they feel they are falling behind. Doing even more work in training than they would if not injured makes sense to them when they feel as if they are playing catch-up.

Planning regeneration days or off days for a rehabilitating athlete is imperative for mental health. Giving the athlete an outlined plan for the week can provide a bit of control over that which can be controlled and gives some ownership of the week's rehabilitation process.

This is powerful during the bridging-the-gap phase, as an athlete struggles with time management when the training or competition schedule is no longer in place.

A rehabilitating athlete often just wants to do more work. However, failing to follow the physiological principle of providing ample recovery for each stress event will not be positive. This often breaks the body down, causes unnecessary fatigue, and increases the risk of re-injury by loading healing tissue too much and too soon.

Incorporating planned off or regeneration days will assist in an athlete's physical recovery process. This process is necessary if the body is to continue repairing the injury damage while also adapting to the revised training load.

This is where the fundamental concepts of the CSCS and other certifications that cover the concepts of strength training come into play. We need to understand the basics to apply physiologically sound methods that help our athletes obtain results and get back on the field.

The following points are applicable to the big picture, but other strength training experts such as Dan John, Michael Boyle, Pavel Tsatsouline, and Mark Verstegen can provide specifics on strength and conditioning topics.

## MUSCLE FIBERS 101

### Type I

The body has different types of muscle fibers that respond to different exercise stimuli. The first are Type I slow-twitch oxidative fibers that create low power output, but have high resistance to fatigue. They are recruited and stimulated with low-intensity aerobic exercise that is often high in volume, light resistance training, and daily activities like walking to get coffee, hiking, or biking to work.

Type I fibers are thin compared with the other fiber types, do not have the same growth potential as Type II variants, and have a small motor neuron. Yet they have a high mitochondrial density and many capillaries because they need a lot of sustained blood flow.

Slow-twitch fibers also have a lower supply of creatine phosphate and lower glycogen content than Type II fibers, but, since their purpose is longer duration activity, they store more triglycerides.

### Type II-A

Next, we have the Type II-A fast-twitch oxidative fibers used during sustained power activities. They are less resistant to fatigue than Type I fibers, but fatigue more slowly than Type II-B due to having moderate glycogen stores.

Like Type I fibers, Type II-A fibers have high myoglobin content and many capillaries and mitochondria. Type II-A fibers have fast contractile speeds and myosin ATPase activity, making them best suited for sports that use both the anaerobic and aerobic glycolysis energy systems and require repeated bursts of rapid activity, such as rugby, basketball, and football. As with the Type II-B variation, Type II-A fibers have a greater growth potential than Type I.[238]

## Type II-B

Finally, we have Type II-B fast-twitch glycolytic fibers, used for high force, power, and speed production, but having low endurance. They are recruited for very short duration high-intensity bursts of power, such as maximal or near-maximal lifts and short sprints.

They do not use oxygen for fuel and have lower capillary and mitochondria density and lower myoglobin content than the other muscle types. Type II-B fibers quickly deplete their high glycogen stores due to fast contraction rates and high power output.

## MUSCLE FIBERS AND BRIDGING THE GAP

Type II-A fibers have the ability to develop characteristics similar to that of Type I fibers or move more toward Type II-B fibers, depending on the training a person undertakes.[239]

This can be detrimental to power-based athletes who are rehabilitating an injury. During the rehab process, movements are often slow and controlled, stimulating those Type II-A fibers to look and act more like Type I fibers.

This leaves fewer fibers functioning on the power side. There is a natural loss of power production and fast movement due to this physiological adaptation.

This is why total-body vibration machines such as the Power Plate® can be useful during the rehab process. Total-body vibration is just that…total-body vibration. The body cannot selectively recruit muscle fibers while standing on a vibration unit—all the muscle fibers will be stimulated.

When performing slow, controlled bodyweight activities on a Power Plate, we can stimulate both Type II-A and Type II-B fibers to improve an athlete's ability to produce power at the physiological level.[240,241]

## THE TIME-UNDER-TENSION CONTINUUM

### Hypertrophy and Applied Functional Hypertrophy

The idea of load and time under tension is one of the fundamental concepts rehabilitation specialists sometimes fail to understand.[242]

Most rehab clinicians love programming three sets of 10 reps; we understand it, we can control the pace, and we can see and coach the movements. It is a comfortable place when working with an athlete.

These types of set and rep schemes often last 20 to 40 seconds per set, and stimulate just enough response from the muscle to gain functional hypertrophy.

We build a bit of muscle, but maybe not exactly what is needed to return to a pre-injury state. This is Applied Functional Hypertrophy, and is often where most rehab specialists live in the time-under-tension continuum.

However, religiously adhering to just three sets of 10—or 5x5, or any other predefined set and rep combination— barely scratches the surface of what an athlete needs before returning to a sport.

A certain number of sets or reps can be used to advance specific performance goals like power application or muscular endurance, but this approach is just one step along the continuum of resistance training.

In a "three sets of 10" session, for example, each set typically lasts between 20 and 40 seconds. This provides just enough time under tension to make strength gains and muscular changes, but not a significant amount.

To help a client regain and perhaps even improve on pre-injury capabilities, we need to advance beyond certain set and rep ranges we are comfortable with prescribing. We need to include time under tension.[243]

Consider this: As a clinician, have you ever helped rehab a person with an ACL injury who did really well? The strength improved, the movement tests were good, the graft healed well, and the person was solid on ligament stress testing.

However, at the end of the rehab, the person had a skinny leg. Even though strong, the leg looked atrophied when compared with the other side. This happens when the rehab did not spend enough time in the hypertrophy phase, which helps people rebound from atrophy caused by injury-related inactivity.[244]

In order to stimulate hypertrophy, muscle must have significant time under tension. Hypertrophy is usually stimulated by sets of nine to 15 reps, with the sets lasting between 40 and 70 seconds. This time under tension is what prompts an increase in the actual size of the muscle fibers, known as myofibril hypertrophy.

## Relative Power

An athlete does not necessarily require greater strength to be more effective in a sport. How far does even an NFL linebacker need to go in the squat rack before getting into the realm of diminishing returns? 400 pounds? 500?

What these athletes often require is more power instead of greater strength, and, more specifically, the ability to apply power on demand in the context of the sport.

Strength is a function of power—this is not to say strength is not important, but it is not everything, particularly on game day. The bottom line is that an athlete needs to express strength as a function of time, also understood to be power application. The two go hand in hand.

We usually train power in one to 10 reps, depending on the activity. When trying to improve an athlete's power output, we think about performing sets of one repetition, no matter how many reps.

We do not think of this as one set of six reps, but six sets of one rep. The athlete brings a very different mindset to the activity with this emphasis, and it often shows up as improved performance.

Power-centric activities typically last less than 10 seconds per set. However, traditional low-rep, high-weight work—such as deadlifts, squats, and Olympic lifts—is not the only kind of power-related training we do.

Power and speed endurance are also important. This shows up when an athlete performs a powerful movement with a higher number of reps than would be used during a dedicated power session, often in sequence with other exercises. The loads will be less than in powerlifting, but the intensity will be higher and the volume greater, helping improve the ability to maintain moderate to high power output longer.

Speed endurance is a variation of this, requiring the athlete to perform several ballistic movements back to back with short, active rest periods between sets.

Power and speed endurance are invaluable in team sports like rugby that require short bursts of intense effort interspersed with periods of lower output. These skill requirements also show up in individual disciplines like cycling, ultra-running, and swimming.

For more on this topic, Brian Mackenzie wrote the book, literally: *Power, Speed, Endurance*.

## Relative Strength

In addition to incorporating power and speed endurance concepts into your training philosophy, it is also important to consider relative strength. As your athletes are returning to sports after injury, you should to pay attention to their strength-to-body-mass ratio, which is often negatively impacted by an injury layoff.

This is particularly true when athletes play a contact sport, as they need to apply strength and power, and to do so against other bodies in motion.

Relative strength is trained in sets of one to five reps that last for less than 20 seconds.

To recap the training terminology in this section:

- ***Hypertrophy***

    *Nine to 15 reps*

    *40–70 seconds per set*

- ***Applied functional hypertrophy***

    *Six to eight reps*

    *20–40 seconds per set*

- ***Relative power***

    *One to 10 or more reps, depending on specificity*

    *Power endurance–capacity of wattage output over time*

- ***Relative strength***

  *One to five reps*

  *Less than 20 seconds per set*

Following these resistance-training guidelines will allow a professional working with an athlete in the return-to-sport phase to dial in the program to address the missing links between rehab and performance.

In particular, these guidelines can significantly help a rehab specialist alter the training stimulus to prepare an athlete to get back into the weight room.

Once there, a strength and conditioning specialist can safely apply these principles.

One of the biggest holes I have seen in the bridging-the-gap philosophy is a rehab specialist who is afraid to move an athlete at different loads and speeds due to a misunderstanding of these concepts. As a result, the athlete shows up in the weight room unprepared for these movements and gets hurt trying to move too much too fast.

There is improved communication when a rehab specialist understands these concepts of time under tension and can describe to the strength coach what is safe or unsafe at a particular point in the process.

This provides the potential for a much better outcome.

## CLINICAL PEARL
### Hypertrophy

- Nine to 15 reps
- 40–70 seconds per set

### Applied functional hypertrophy

- Six to eight reps
- 20–40 seconds per set

### Relative power

- One to 10 or more reps, depending on specificity
- Power endurance—capacity of wattage output over time

### Relative strength

- One to five reps
- Less than 20 seconds per set

## EXERCISE MODALITIES AND APPLICATION

When prescribing resistance-training activities, we have a variety of modalities in our toolbox. Whatever modality we use, it is simply a tool.

We use tools to express our philosophy of training. They do not dictate our philosophy of training. A dumbbell, a machine, a TRX® Suspension Trainer, a kettlebell, or a medicine ball are all tools we use to express a philosophy. The use of any one of them is not a philosophy in and of itself.

Free weights allow increased range of motion and require more internal stability than machine-based lifts. Depending on positioning, they also involve greater proprioception, positional competence, and balance from the athlete.

The idea of free weights is sometimes used in a limiting way, but these can include dumbbells, barbells, kettlebells, and any other tool that does not fix the athlete into a certain position the way a machine does.

Machines limit range of motion and take away the internal stability requirement by providing the external stability of the machine. This potentially allows people to move higher loads because of this additional external stability.

Some would say this is good, as equipment such as a leg press provides the body with an over-stimulus to push more mass, therefore stimulating relative strength gains.

However, others argue that strength without the internal ability to stabilize the forces is not only unnecessary and inapplicable to the sports field, but is also dangerous.

Still, machines can come in handy in our bridging-the-gap process when we have an athlete who is post surgical or injured and unable to use an extremity. With a machine, we might be able to safely introduce strength training without worrying about an athlete getting hurt trying to control a free weight.

There is a place for every exercise modality. The choice should be left to the professional to decide when and how these tools are applied during the rehab-to-performance continuum, just as when factoring in other disciplines such as Pilates or yoga.

## EXERCISE SELECTION VOCABULARY

In recent years, strength and conditioning paradigms have moved away from training muscles and body parts and toward training movements. There is a time and place for individual muscle training, specifically early in the post-injury rehab process and certainly with post-operative athletes.

After an acute injury or surgery, the body needs to "reconnect" with that area. This is where the neuromuscular connections forged by a more isolative exercise can have value.

However, as the person moves through the rehab continuum and gets closer to a return to competition, coordinated movements that involve sequencing multiple muscle groups are more valuable. [245]

When putting this continuum into action at EXOS, we created a system of communication that is easy for the strength and conditioning and specialties to use. It was one of the most significant things we did to facilitate the process.

In discussions about athletes who were returning to play, Ken Croner, then a strength coach with EXOS and currently the co-owner of Munster Sports Performance, and I as the PT would often have a recurring discussion.

Ken: "Can he do this exercise?"

Me: "No."

Ken: "What about this exercise?"

Me: "Yes."

Ken: "How about this one?"

Me: "No."

This conversation would last until we covered every item in the training program to determine what the athlete could do. Ken would then write a new workout, bring it back for consideration, and the process would begin again.

All of the coaches and PTs at EXOS knew this was an inefficient process. We needed to develop a common language, one in which all exercises could be categorized for more efficient communication between the health care practitioner and the strength coach.

We developed the following terms about 12 years ago—they may or may not have been in use before that. At the time, they were new to me, and we had enough discussion around them to let me know they were most likely not mainstream terms at the time.

Either way, this lexicon was new to our system and proved to be highly beneficial in helping athletes move from the acute post-injury phase, through retraining, and all the way back to competition.

The categories we applied included:

## Upper-body push and pull

- *Horizontal or vertical*
- *Rotational*
- *Unilateral, alternating, or bilateral*

## Lower-body push and pull

- *Single leg or double leg*
- *Hip dominant or knee dominant*
- *Rotational*

## Propulsive and stabilization

- *Rotational movements*

## CLINICAL PEARL
### MOVEMENT TYPES

### Upper-Body Push and Pull

- Horizontal or vertical

- Rotational

- Unilateral, alternating, or bilateral

### Lower-Body Push and Pull

- Single leg or double leg

- Hip dominant or knee dominant

### Rotational

- Propulsive and stabilization

## USING THE UPPER-BODY CATEGORY

Are you pushing the load away from you or are you pulling it toward you? Are you doing this in a manner that makes the load parallel or perpendicular to the body—it is vertical or horizontal? Are you doing the movement with one arm, both arms at the same time, or are you alternating moving the arms left to right?

That description pretty much covers all upper-body movements, while recognizing there is a rotational component to movement as well. A pullup is a vertical pull in which the load is parallel to the body. A shoulder press is a vertical push—the load is parallel to the body. A pushup is a push where the load is perpendicular to the body, and so on.

With this simple language, a PT can say to a strength coach, "The player who has shoulder impingement can perform all upper-body horizontal pulling and external rotation activities."

This means the athlete can do any row variation the coach can devise in this plane of motion, without needing to go into a jargon-heavy explanation about the athlete's shoulder joint, or without the strength coach explaining every possible implement in the weight room.

One arm, two arms, half-kneeling on a bench—it does not matter. The coach can choose the tools to express the program based on which athlete is doing the work. While effectively improving a player's strength and power, we have peace of mind, knowing the athlete whose health we are responsible for is training safely and not irritating the injured area.

As we move along the continuum and a player gets closer to clearance for play, we progress to vertical pulling, then horizontal pushing and internal rotation.

The last progression for an athlete is usually overhead pushing. In fact, that category might never be introduced, based on the player's training or chronological age, injury history, physical limitations, and current playing status.

The strength coach and medical staff all know what kind of upper-body training is appropriate at the time, thanks to this use of clearly defined terminology.

## USING THE LOWER-BODY CATEGORY

Lower-body pushing and pulling can get a bit confusing, as some people define these differently. At that time at Athletes' Performance, we evaluated pushing or pulling relating to the center of gravity. Are you pushing the mass away from your center of gravity or are you pulling the mass toward it?

In this definition, a pushing activity would be a squat or any squat variation, such as a leg press or pistol. A pulling activity would be a deadlift-type activity.

The next question: Are you doing this with two legs on the ground or a single leg? Is this movement knee dominant, as in a squat or hamstring curl, or it is hip dominant like a Romanian deadlift?

If an athlete has anterior knee pain, we might use a hip-dominant lower-body activity. We might start with pulling hip movements and then progress to pushing exercises.

When coming off an acute injury, we might do everything on two legs, eventually progressing to single-leg variations. We might only do single-leg variations on the uninjured side.

With this system, the strength and conditioning coach has a simple mandate for each athlete's training, without having to first run every variation by the medical staff, who may not be up to speed on all the available training modalities.

## PROPULSIVE VERSUS STABILIZING ROTATIONAL ACTIVITIES

We define stabilization activities for the core to include those activities that require the athlete to stabilize against a rotational force.

This is in contrast to propulsive exercises, which require people to move and rotate through the hips, introducing an element of kinetic linking into the activity. From a rehabilitation standpoint, we typically start with stabilization movements and progress to propulsive drills.

For example, you are probably familiar with Gray Cook's chop and lift activities.

A lift is a stabilization exercise, as the athlete is trying to stabilize the trunk against a rotational force.

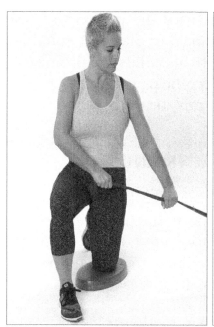 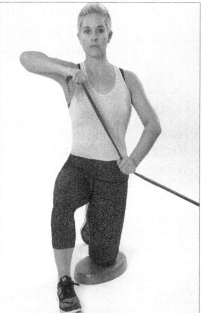 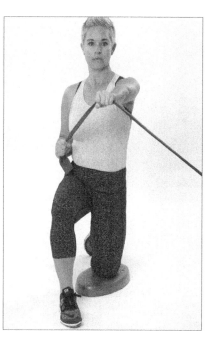

**Photos 9.1a–9.1c—Stability Lift**

*In this exercise, the athlete can have a variety of lower-body positions such as tall kneel, half kneel, or split stance to challenge balance by altering the base of support.*

*The upper body does a single-arm upright rowing motion with the outside arm, and then a push movement with the inside arm. No rotation is allowed in the torso, as the body is trying to stabilize against rotational forces.*

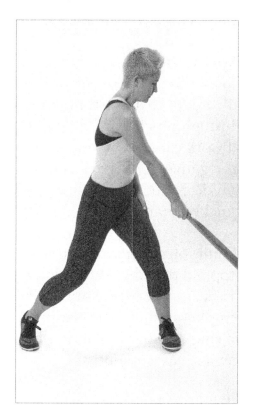

**Photo 9.2—Rotational Row, Start Position**

*In this exercise, the goal of the movement is general rotation. Although stability is still required through the lumbar spine, rotation is allowed at the shoulders, thoracic spine, hips, and lower extremity.*

*The athlete is attempting to produce rotational movement, starting from this position of a rotated athletic base.*

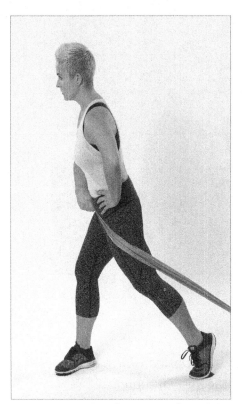

**Photo 9.3—Rotational Row, End Position**

*The end position of the exercise can have a variety of upper-extremity positions, such as single arm to opposite hip as shown here or two hands starting low and ending in an overhead pushing movement. The back leg will have elements of external rotation and extension, while the forward leg will have elements of internal rotation.*

A stability lift is a stability exercise—the athlete is moving the upper extremity while preventing rotation in the trunk.

A rotational row is a propulsive exercise. The athlete is combining rotational forces at the upper extremity, thoracic spine, and hips on a neutral lumbar spine.

The ability to stabilize against a rotational force, as well as the ability to produce a rotational force are key movements an athlete returning to play will need to master. This helps the person to resist forces on the field of play that could be harmful, and the ability to produce a rotational force helps create the power necessary for athletic movement.

## ADDITIONAL TRAINING VARIABLES

There are dozens of possible training variables, but we are going to focus on those that pertain to athlete performance and health.

**Training age** is not the same as chronological age. A 35-year-old who has never trained is a novice trainee. A 22-year-old who is a Division I collegiate athlete is most likely an intermediate or even an experienced trainee. From a movement prescription standpoint, you need to consider training age when determining other programming variables, such as frequency, density, volume, and intensity.[246]

Novice trainees typically need to develop all physical attributes. They can usually adapt to most stimulation and learn through repetition. Though their general work capacity is low, do not look at as a negative. This gives you something to build on; they will often progress more quickly than a highly trained athlete.

Think of a time in your life when you stopped training. When you got back on track, you were probably exhausted by a simple workout. The beauty of being out of shape is that it does not take much to get a great workout.

People respond to nearly any stimulus when undertrained.

An intermediate trainee needs to build the racecar for the competition. With these people, you need to apply more advanced concepts of periodization to ensure the athlete responds to the stimulus. You may also need to develop specific attributes using varied stimulation, such as frequently changing the programming so the body does not plateau the way it does when the stimulus stays the same.

An advanced trainee is like fine-tuning a racecar. These people are adding horse power to movement patterns—which requires even better brakes—or gaining greater ability to decelerate. An advanced trainee needs very specific training parameters. Stimuli may change often, as they will quickly adapt to new training variables.

**Training volume** is the amount of training completed or the total amount of work done, such as time or distance. This could be a 5K run performed continuously or 1,500 meters broken up into 150-meter intervals with active rest between each interval.

**Training intensity** tells us how strenuous the training is, typically measured as a percentage of a known maximum. For example, a clean and jerk session might be considered 95 percent of the athlete's intensity capacity.

**Training frequency** refers to how often the training stress is applied.

**Training density** typically suggests how much work is performed in a certain period, such as in an *As Many Rounds as Possible* workout.

A novice trainee might only train two or three times per week, using lower loads to learn the movements, and the workout may take an hour to perform.

An intermediate trainee could do that same workout four or five times per week, with higher loads and at various speeds. It might only take 45 minutes to do the more aggressive workout.

In the second example, the training frequency, intensity, and density have all increased, while the general volume of the single training session might be the same. If you add more exercises to the second workout, you have also increased the volume.

Volume, intensity, density, and frequency provide us with simple ways to alter programming based on each athlete's individual needs and abilities, as well as the ultimate return-to-play needs.

## PERIODIZATION

In the simplest terms, periodization is the manipulation of training stress over a period to produce a desired outcome.[247] It consists of several cycles over the course of the training year. Macrocycles are periods of the year and comprise several blocks of mesocycles.

Each mesocycle aims to achieve certain objectives and is made up of several microcycles, each of which generally lasts between five and 14 days. Several training days make up a microcycle, and several microcycles comprise a mesocycle.

A physical therapist in a traditional setting usually does not work with a patient long enough to see the person all the way through a full macrocycle. However, the rehab process itself might be considered a mesocycle.

It is important for the clinician to understand these strength and conditioning concepts to be able to work well with other sports-medicine professionals. This will help the entire care team create an actionable plan to help the athlete return to competition at full capacity, as soon as possible, but without increasing the risk of re-injury.

## Rehab Periodization

The principles of periodization need not be confined to programming an athlete's training. Periodization can also be applied to the various stages of rehabilitation as we bridge this gap between the two.[248] We can think of rehab as being a mesocycle, with a goal of completing rehab. Microcycles are the smaller chunks of activity along the way.

For example, if someone is post-operative, the first microcycle goal could be to regain full range of motion. The second microcycle might focus on balance and proprioception. The third microcycle could concentrate on neuromuscular control.

This does not mean each microcycle can only focus on one physical attribute. There are many ways to periodize a rehabilitation program, such as the following concepts.

### Linear

In this model, we use periodic sequencing to train one physical quality after another. We could work on range of motion first, then balance and proprioception, and then psychomotor control and strength.

Although every rehab may have a different linear progression based on the patient's needs, most clinicians agree that regaining necessary motion is the priority. Strength and balance are addressed at any point, but range of motion must be regained early to prevent a slew of other issues later in the rehab process.

### Concurrent

During concurrent training, we address several competing physical qualities in one mesocycle. Strength and endurance might be viewed as "competing" from a physiological standpoint, and could be part of a concurrent training program.[249]

A large volume of endurance training has a negative impact on strength gains, while long-duration, lower-output work is only minimally affected by the introduction of strength training. If you are working with a marathoner, introducing strength activities should have minimal effect on endurance qualities.[250]

However, when training a football player or someone who does not often function aerobically, performing long-duration, low-load activities can negatively impact strength and power gains.

It is important to understand this idea: Strength and power training can greatly assist endurance athletes, while endurance training can negatively impact those who need more power.

In untrained people, the interference effect is minimal. However, in moderately or highly trained athletes, concurrent training affects the rate of force development or power more significantly than absolute strength.[251]

## Conjugate

With conjugated programming, we are training several complementary qualities in one mesocycle. Examples might include strength and power, or somatosensory control and psychomotor control.

From a rehab perspective, we certainly can work on getting the right muscle to fire at the right time, while at the same time working to improve balance and proprioception for a given joint. Working on one of these would not interfere with the progress of the other. Therefore, these would be considered conjugated programming.

## Concentrated

Concentrated training involves short periods of high training stress aimed at improving a single physical quality. We often use this method as an athlete is closing in on the strength training aspect of rehab.

For example, if an athlete is getting stiff at an injured joint, the clinician may have concerns that gaining this range of motion will only get more difficult or even impossible if left alone.

The clinician may decide that one or two weeks are needed to dedicate every effort into regaining that active or passive range of motion back in the joint. All other concerns of strength or balance might be on hold until the athlete is able to restore the natural range of motion in the joint.

We can use also *blocks*, which are sequential chunks of concentrated mesocycles.

When an athlete is nearing return to competition, we might need to taper the program. This is a rapid reduction in volume or intensity to facilitate supercompensation before competition.

There might be no tapering phase or might be used exclusively when bridging the gap from rehab to performance. Since the athlete is usually progressing slowly and building up to the return-to-competition phase, we may only use a brief rest period of a day versus a true tapering prior to returning to competition.

Finally, we have the pre-competition phase, which comes at the end of the continuum, right before the athlete returns to competition.

For example, if a baseball player plays in AAA games for several nights, the taper might simply be one day off for travel before joining the big league club to play the following day.

When discussing this with the team manager, you might decide it is best that the athlete only returns to competition for a few innings instead of an entire game.

This decrease in volume, along with a rise in intensity, may suffice as the athlete's taper prior to return to full competition.

This concept is planned in conjunction with the strength and conditioning specialist. Each situation needs to be evaluated by everyone involved in the care continuum. This way you can devise an appropriate return-to-sport plan that prepares the athlete for the return and safeguards longer-term health.

## SUMMARY

Strength is the fundamental building block to power. Ultimately, an athlete will need to be able to move at varying loads and speeds to return to competition. Preparing an athlete to do this is paramount when bridging the gap from rehab to performance. Strength and conditioning coaches can be significant resources to health care professionals who are not accustomed to applying these concepts to their rehabilitation programs.

It will benefit your athletes as they prepare to return to play if you understand strength-training principles and know how to safely apply them to your rehabilitation programs.

# CHAPTER TEN
## FUNDAMENTAL ADVANCEMENT

Now it is time to keep the client moving forward toward competitive readiness. We have identified and treated a pain generator, restored range of motion and basic strength to the affected motion segment, retrained the psychomotor system, addressed somatosensory influences, and focused on the total-body concepts of strength and power development.

The next stage in the rehab continuum is to reestablish athletic movement capabilities diminished by the traumatic injury or surgery, and for clients suffering from chronic issues.

To kick-start an athlete's fundamental advancement, we need to pull from our strength and conditioning models. It is up to you whether to follow EXOS, Michael Boyle's CFSC, standard ACSM, CSCS formulas, or any of the other leading schools.

Power development using kettlebell training, Olympic lifting, or any other specialization helps our clients get back on the field, but you need to consider their overall wellbeing, training age, your available equipment, and more. It does not matter which tool you use, as long as it delivers results within the continuum of care.

In this penultimate stage of the bridging-the-gap model, we focus on universal movements and athletic competencies that are often diminished in the wake of an injury.

Once we have worked with clients on fundamental-advancement exercises and they show no ill effects, it will time to move into the final phase, the advanced performance discussed in Chapter Eleven. That is the point where we concentrate on sharpening sport-specific skills before clearance to return to a full practice or playing schedule.

## DIRECTION AND PLANES OF MOTION

Movement can be broken up and categorized according to the direction of travel. When approaching this from a high level, we move linearly, laterally, rotationally, up, or down.

These categories can then be further broken down to introduce the patterns to someone who is beginning to move at various speeds following injury.

Before we add speed or power to a movement, the client must have the foundational building blocks of strength to accept that training. Fundamental performance sets the foundation of strength and is where we begin to introduce the concepts of moving at various loads and speeds so the athlete can apply these concepts to foundational athletic movement.

Bridging the gap from rehab to performance requires specific and full understanding of each of the following movement patterns, which allows us to teach in pieces to build into a whole.

## LINEAR MOVEMENT

Linear movement can be defined as moving in the sagittal plane in relation to oneself. That movement can be forward or backward and can cover a short distance of under 10 yards or a longer distance. This can be broken up into four distinct subsections:

- *Acceleration*

- *Absolute speed*

- *Deceleration*

- *Backpedaling*

## ACCELERATION

When you are accelerating at the start of a 100-meter sprint, you are in a total-body lean, with great sprinters getting close to a 45-degree angle to the ground as they drive out of the blocks and get up to speed. All of the power in the legs is driving down and back, in a piston-like action to propel the body forward as opposed to falling forward.

This application of all-out speed is hard enough to master for a healthy athlete and is even more difficult for those recovering from an injury.

Early in my career at Athletes' Performance as I was beginning to learn, understand, and dissect these movement patterns, we were working with several athletes on the track, one of whom was a hockey player.

Despite the fact that he performed his athletic skill on ice, he still benefited from strength and conditioning work off the rink; running was part of his workout that day. Observing him do some of the drills demonstrated how difficult it can be to apply strength and power to acceleration without losing body control.

The coach used a drill that started with the athlete lying on his stomach. On the coach's command, the hockey player was to get up as fast as he could and begin sprinting for 10 to 20 yards.

The athlete was on his stomach with his hands at shoulder level, waiting for the coach's cue. When the coach yelled "Go!" he surged with all his might, took about four steps and unceremoniously face-planted on the track.

Given that he was a driven athlete who was motivated to improve, nothing could deter him from getting the drill right, not even embarrassment or abrasions from collapsing on the track.

Back to the start for another go, the same thing happened: He face-planted within four steps. A third attempt yielded the same results.

It was not until the fourth try that the hockey player finally figured out he was not on ice. He could not use the same lower-body strategy of hip extension at about 45 degrees behind him as he did to generate speed on the ice. Instead, he had to drive down and back, directly behind him to thrust himself forward.

According to Newton's third law, every action has an equal and opposite reaction. You cannot inappropriately put force into the ground and expect the ground to return an equal and meaningful force.

Acceleration is all about angles and force application. When you are working with an athlete, you need to understand this force application and institute activities designed to help the client do this in an efficient manner.

## The Components of Acceleration

While there are a lot of biomechanical subtleties involved, acceleration is comprised of four main aspects:

- *Body position–total-body lean*

- *Leg action*

- *Arm action*

- *Ankle dorsiflexion*

### Body Position—Total-Body Lean

Total-body lean is what propels us forward as we apply force toward the ground. As described in the hockey player example, every action has an equal and opposite reaction.

If you are standing upright and apply force into the ground, you will go upward in a jump. In contrast, if in a total-body lean you apply a force directly behind, you propel forward.

However, body lean can only go so far before the center of gravity and joint alignment becomes detrimental to balance. If you get too far forward and your legs drive out to the side, you will fall flat on your face like that hockey player.

Total-body lean means exactly that… total-body lean. It does not imply bending forward at the waist while the legs remain straight up and down. Look at the total-body lean shown in Photo 10.1.

### Leg Action

The leg action in this total-body lean must be piston-like to effectively accelerate. Imagine pistons in a car, driving up and down. This is how our legs need to drive into the ground to send ourselves forward.

Another key component of leg action is the concept of hip separation. Think of bouncing a basketball. If you bounce the ball lightly down by your lower leg, not much force is produced. However, if you take that basketball overhead and then slam it into the ground, you will get an equal and opposite reaction, sending the ball high into the air.

The same principles apply to hip separation. If you barely lift your leg off the ground, you will not have much force to put into the ground; the return of your energy investment will be low for your next stride.

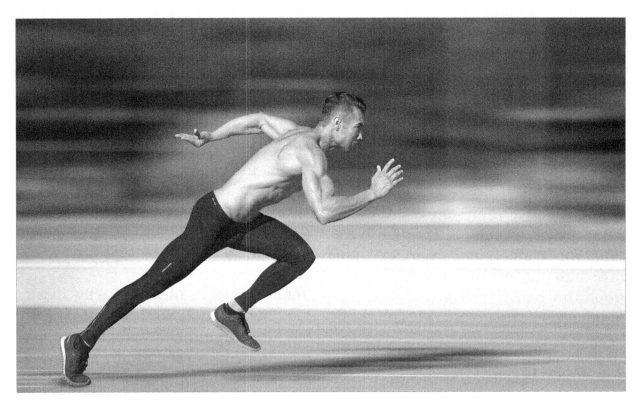

**Photo 10.1—Acceleration**

*When looking at this picture, you can easily see all elements of acceleration in this athlete's form.*

*He has total-body lean, meaning he is not flexed at his hips, but is in a complete lean of his entire body toward his target. His legs are driving down and back in a piston-like action to propel him forward.*

*His elbows are bent and he is using his shoulders to drive back and create momentum forward; his lead ankle is dorsiflexed, ready to be driven down into the ground for forward motion.*

*This is an excellent real-life example of acceleration captured in a single instant.*

Yet if you lift your leg up to 90 degrees and then drive it into the ground, you will get a larger return for your effort. This is like a sprinter flying down the track, trying to exert as much power as physically possible into each stride.

However, just as with body lean, there is a limit to how high up the leg drive should originate. If you bring your leg up so high that you compromise the position of the low back, you will decrease the stability of the trunk, which is your base. That will affect balance as well as the energy return when you start to make compensations in form to gain artificial stability. There is a fine line in proper hip separation.

It is also a crucial factor to ensure optimal hip mobility in your clients. Your athletes will not be able to generate maximum acceleration force when tight in the anterior hip, which limits extension, or in the posterior hip, limiting flexion.

## Arm Action

Arm action is the third key to reaching full acceleration potential. As we do not perform any movement skill in isolation, arm action will largely dictate leg action. Assuming we have the requisite mobility and motor control in the hips and legs, generating powerful arm action will encourage the legs to follow suit.

Let us test this: Sit on the ground with your legs stretched out in front of you. Bend your elbows to 90 degrees. Now, drive your elbows reciprocally back as hard and as fast as you can. What should happen is that your butt bounces off the ground as you are literally moving your body with the action of your arms.

However, if you lose the elbow angle, you will slam your hand into the ground and no force will be created. If you move your arms slowly, you will not bounce. Drive really hard with just your right arm with your left arm still and you might begin to turn.

Arm action is important when teaching the legs what to do while running. In the example of the hockey player, the coach told him to think about his arms and to drive them back as hard as he could. This simple cue is what cleared up his leg action and prevented more humiliating and painful face plants.

## Ankle Dorsiflexion

The final key to acceleration is ankle dorsiflexion, where we have a couple of things to consider. When the ankle is dorsiflexed, it is in a closed-packed position, meaning there is good bony congruency of the joint. When the ankle is plantar flexed, the talus rolls forward out of the mortise and we leave stability up to the ligaments, capsule, and skin of the joint.

In reverse, for stability when the ankle is dorsiflexed, we rely on the bony fit of the talus in the mortsie—the arch formed at the anterior ankle by the tibia and fibula.

It is much better to try to produce power from a stable base—power requires a foundation from which to produce force. When it comes to biomechanics, joint stability is what provides this base.

As we covered in the motion-segment chapter beginning on page 65, joint centration is not only crucial for quality power transmission, but also to prevent structural damage.

Secondly, when the ankle is dorsiflexed, it places the contractile tissues of the ankle plantar flexors on stretch. This allows us to almost spring off the tissue.

If the ankle is plantar flexed and we land on the forefoot, we have to absorb force by allowing the heel to lower to the ground. Then we have to reproduce this force to propel us forward.

If the ankle is dorsiflexed and the arches of the feet are not compromised, we simply spring off the forefoot, bringing the leg back into flexion to begin the next cycle of reciprocal motion.

## WALL DRILLS

From a rehabilitative standpoint and a fundamental-advancement perspective, the wall drills we used at Athletes' Performance are invaluable in my practice. Using the wall to teach body angle, hip separation, leg action, and ankle dorsiflexion provides a huge lesson in breaking down the acceleration movement pattern.

Here are a few examples.

**Photo 10.2—Wall Hold** *(at right)*

*For a select period, the athlete will hold all aspects of acceleration other than arm action. For rehab professionals, this is your progression of a plank—it is basically an acceleration-position plank.*

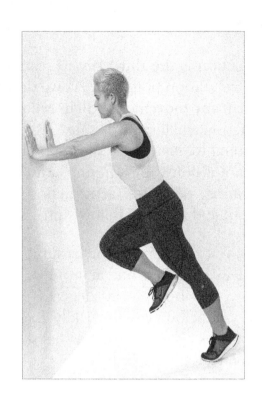

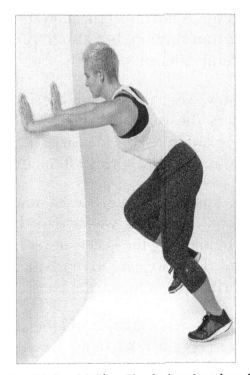

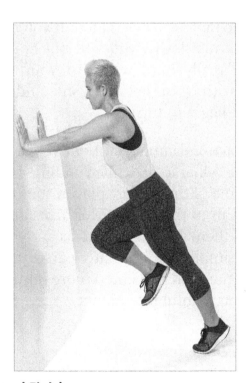

**Photos 10.3a–10.3b—Single-Leg Load and Lift, Start and Finish**

*This is a single-leg squat variation in an acceleration position. The emphasis should be on the power movement toward the wall.*

In this progression, the athlete has both feet off the ground at one point, for the first time. The athlete starts in the holding position and drives down one leg, thinking about it causing the other leg to come up to the same position.

*Triple exchange (not pictured):* This is the same exercise as the single exchange, except the legs are exchanged three times. The biggest mistake athletes make on this is short stepping the middle step—not allowing full hip separation to occur.

*Exchange for time (not pictured):* Use this exchange exercise for time instead of reps—five seconds, 10 seconds, or longer.

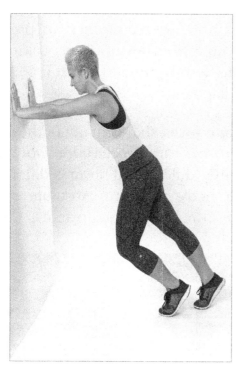

**Photo 10.4—Up Down**

*The athlete drops the foot to the position indicated and rebounds it back to the starting position.*

*The biggest mistake people make with this is putting too little emphasis on the downward motion and too much emphasis on the lifting portion. When cueing this exercise, instruct the athlete to drive the foot into the ground and let it bounce back to the original position, like a basketball.*

*When dribbling, we do not think about how the basketball travels from the ground back to the hand, only from the hand to the ground. Somehow it shows back up in the hand as a result of the driving force downward.*

*Single Exchange (not pictured):* In this exercise, the athlete begins in the same position as in Photo 10.2. The leg is driven into the ground, and at the same time, the opposite leg is coming into the flexed position.

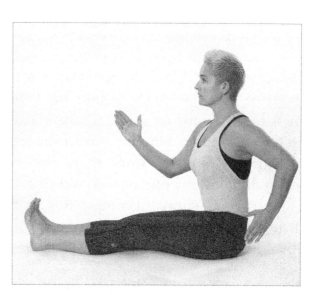

**Photo 10.5—Arm Action**

*The legs are extended straight as the athlete sits on the ground with the elbows bent to 90 degrees. The elbows drive backward for time, hard and fast, to "bounce" the athlete off the ground.*

Acceleration is a fundamental athletic movement for most athletes participating in land-based, movement-centric sports.

Understanding the components of acceleration and how to coach these elements in parts and eventually combining them into the whole movement is necessary for rehab professionals and performance professionals alike.

## ABSOLUTE SPEED

Absolute speed typically occurs when an athlete is running greater than 10 to 15 yards. In the context of a sport, not all athletes need absolute speed.

During my time working with athletes preparing for the NFL Combine, I hated the week we introduced absolute speed to the offensive linemen because many of them had not run more than 10 yards for a very long time.

However, this skill is necessary for them to run the 40-yard dash held in such high regard as a testing standard at the Combine. Despite proper tissue preparation and skill work, there would inevitably be someone who would strain a hamstring, simply because the soft tissues were not ready for the rigors of absolute speed work.

As a comparison, imagine the first time you tried to perform a handstand. Unless you had a gymnastics background, that probably did not go so well. No matter how strong the core and upper body, the first time most people do a handstand, they fail to get the legs high enough over the body. If they do get their legs up, they usually go too far over the torso, causing a tumble to the side or over the top of their hands.

It is the same with absolute speed. If the tissues are not accustomed to producing power from an upright position, it is going to take time to reach a person's athletic potential.

Absolute speed shares many of the components of other acceleration work, but is slightly different. The first difference is the body position. Absolute speed requires the body to be upright.

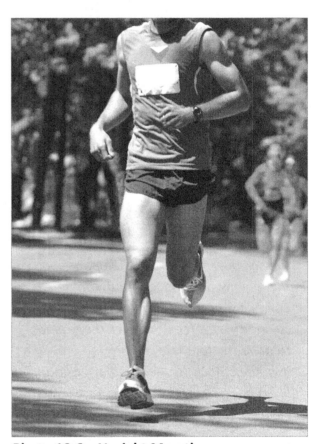

**Photo 10.6—Upright Marathoner**

*Compare the body position of the marathon runner above with the sprinter below. Notice how the body position here is more upright and the legs are functioning in move of a cyclical fashion. The arm action and the need for ankle dorsiflexion remain the same.*

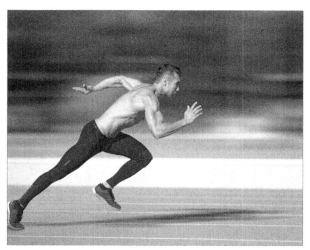

**Photo 10.7— Sprinter**

*Notice the postural differences from someone who is in an acceleration position and in an absolute speed position shown in Photo 10.6. The two postures and leg actions are very different, while the foot action and arm action are similar.*

*"Return the athlete to running" is not a sufficient goal. As professionals working with athletes to bridge the gap from rehab to performance, we must know the type of running they need in their sports and select the exercise progressions accordingly.*

Think of marathoners and consider the uprightness of position. They are not leaning far forward at the waist, or in a total-body lean as in sprinting. They are upright or very close to it.

You will see another difference in the leg action. Although hip separation is still an important concept in generating absolute speed, leg action is cyclical instead of piston-like, with the legs moving in a more bicycle-type fashion. During this cyclical motion, the heel stays close to the thigh for a quick leg recovery.

To better absorb this, stand up and put all of your weight on one leg. Now take the unweighted leg and begin to swing it back and forth from front to back as fast as you can.

Next, bend your knee until your heel is touching your butt and do the same swinging motion as fast as you can. With the heel touching your butt, you have a much shorter lever to move.

A shorter lever means a faster motion and therefore faster speed. This shows how important heel recovery contributes to leg action when teaching absolute speed.

Just like acceleration, we can use the wall to practice and coach the components of absolute speed with the athletes. Wall drills are a big part of my practice in bridging the gap from rehab to performance when introducing movement patterns back into the athletes' training regimes.

A few examples follow on the next page.

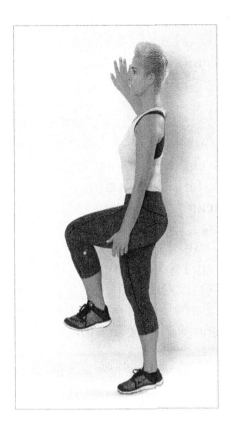

**Photo 10.8—Wall Hold Variation** *(at left)*

*The athlete holds the posture pictured for a select amount of time. Cue to keep the weight on the stance leg focused on the front part of the foot, using the idea that you could slide a piece of paper under the heel as a visual for the client.*

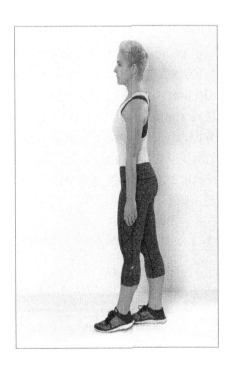 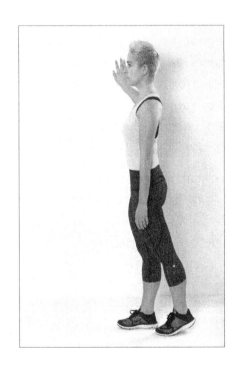

**Photos 10.9a and 10.9b—One Cycle, Midpoint**

*The athlete "claws" down to the ground and with a quick heel recovery in mind, slides the metatarsal heads across the ground until getting some amount of hip extension that does not compromise the lumbar spine position.*

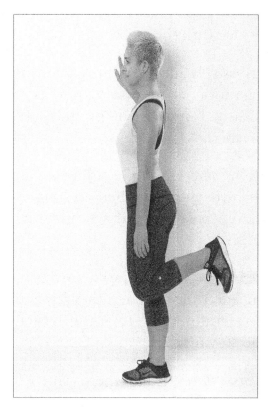

**Photo 10.10—One Cycle, Finish**

*The athlete then brings heel to butt and, keeping the leg tight in maximal knee flexion. The athlete then brings the knee forward and the hip back to the starting position as shown in Photo 10.8.*

*Two cycles:* Once the athlete is able to perform one cycle with some speed, do two or more cycles with speed, being careful not to compromise the lumbar spine position, which is a common compensatory pattern.

## DECELERATION

There is no doubt that as an expression of explosive power and speed, acceleration carries some injury risk due to the great forces applied to soft tissues, connective tissues, and joints. Yet, it is arguable that more injuries occur during the deceleration that follows.

Consider basketball or volleyball. We do not see many injuries resulting from a player leaping up to dunk or spike, but rather from the off-axis impact of an awkward landing.

It is the same with sprinting in a rugby, soccer, or American football game. Certainly, muscle strains can occur while an athlete is getting up to speed; however, it is often slowing down or during a transition—like changing direction or going from sprinting to jumping—that seems to lead to more injured athletes.

The challenges with deceleration include dynamic stabilization of a rapidly moving body and absorbing the force created by the acceleration.

Alternatively, in the case of a movement transition, think of creating force, absorbing it, and then creating it again. This can involve force generation and management in multiple planes and directions, which often gives athletes trouble from an injury perspective.

We have speed and strength and conditioning coaches focused on building big physical engines, but it is also necessary to spend time developing the requisite brakes to slow these racecars down.[252]

When people are coming back from injuries, the ability to dynamically stabilize is compromised. It is easy to guess what happens when we add to this the components of speed, power, explosiveness, and swift directional changes.

It is our job in the rehab continuum to enhance the ability to stabilize, absorb force, and manage the demands of quick transitions so the athletes can produce force at game speed.

As with other exercises in this chapter, deceleration drills should be progressively layered so they become increasingly demanding. Keep the volume low and provide plenty of rest to ensure the muscles and fascia have ample time to recover before the next stimulus.

As your athlete progresses without problems, add a little more volume and increase the density by reducing the active rest periods. Acceleration and deceleration are very taxing and can be trained two or at the most three sessions per week.

## Deceleration Drills

A progressing athlete will have to learn how to decelerate at the same time as relearning to accelerate. As the athlete is gaining neuromotor control, strength, and power, you should introduce deceleration progressions at the same time.

This is often unconscious, as the athlete will naturally slow down the movement after a repetition is complete.

Nevertheless, having a more structured introduction, discussion, and progression of deceleration will benefit your athletes as they progress in the bridging-the-gap continuum.

We could argue that deceleration should be developed prior to maximum power or acceleration. The clinical art of how we progress athletes remains up for

debate. These phases may take several weeks to work through.

Progressively increasing the intensity of deceleration is necessary, just as with every other movement progression we prescribe.

*Phase one*: Have the athletes run 40 yards and give them as long as they need to slow down after the finish.

*Phase two*: Repeat the 40-yard run, but this time tell them they have to decelerate by the time they reach the 60-yard line.

*Phase three*: Have them run 40 yards a third time and reduce the deceleration window to 10 yards. Rest for two minutes.

*Phase four*: For the fourth segment, ask them to come to a halt within five yards of finishing the 40-yard sprint.

*Phase five*: After the 40-yard dash, have the athletes stop "on a dime" with no window.

*Phase six:* After the 40-yard dash, have the athlete stop on a dime, and then as quickly as possible run for 10 yards to the left or right.

If you are working in a sporting environment that does not have lines such as those of a football field, you can either use cones to mark the distances or use the game's natural markers, like bases in baseball or the halfway line and 18-yard penalty box in soccer.

### Deceleration Jumping Drill

Athletes should learn how to land before learning how to jump up. However, gravity makes this a challenge. In order to break this process down, try the following progression:

*Phase one*: Have the athlete stand on a 12-inch box with the feet shoulder width apart and then drop down and land on both feet.

Be sure the weight is not in the heels, but more toward the front of the foot near the metatarsal heads. The landing should be soft, absorbing force at the foot, ankle, knees, and hips.

*Phase two*: Repeat the drill using a 16-inch box.

*Phase three*: Increase the drop height as needed for the athlete's sport.

*Phase four*: Once the athlete lands, cue to immediately explode upward into a vertical jump, landing with the proper biomechanics demonstrated in the first three steps.

### Upper-Extremity Deceleration Drill

Sports that involve throwing, catching, and wielding a tool like a bat or a racquet require athletes to decelerate the upper body at the end of the movement. Without this, a pitcher would go flying off the mound, a tennis player would spin around, and a quarterback would end up with his face in the dirt.

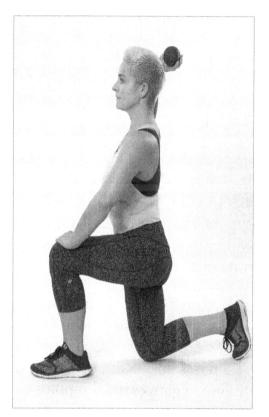

**Photo 10.11—Half-Kneeling Throwing Deceleration**

*In the half-kneeling position, the athlete looks ahead, while the clinician throws the ball from behind. The athlete attempts to catch the ball in midair as it comes over the shoulder, and slows it down on the follow-through.*

*As a progression, the athlete can throw it back over the shoulder towards the clinician, implementing plyometric principles for the upper extremity.*

If you have the required knowledge, you can create sport-specific drills for your athletes. If not, here is a more generic idea that is effective for players returning from injury in many sports.

*Step one*: Have the player get into a half-kneeling position.

*Step two*: Stand a few feet behind and throw a medicine ball over the person's head.

*Step three*: The athlete will track the flight of the ball, catch it, and decelerate the arms to stop the tip forward.

*Step four*: Repeat the drill, but this time, have the person throw it back to you. This introduces concepts of the stretch-shorten cycle plyometrics, which we will cover on page 223.

A large part of dynamic stabilization is the ability to control eccentric muscular contraction. For this, we also incorporate exercises like Romanian deadlifts and pullup negatives that emphasize this type of contraction.

## BACKPEDALING

Backpedaling is a movement type that does not fall into the usual categories. It is not typically included with linear motion drills, even though it clearly is one, nor is it lumped with acceleration or deceleration, despite including elements of both.

Backpedaling is not taken into account when thinking about concentric or eccentric contraction work, though it requires competence in each. As clinicians and performance coaches, many in our professions have focused on getting clients back to running as a measure of readiness, without giving backpedaling a second thought.

Despite being hard to categorize, there is a time in most sports in which backpedaling is required. This might be a quarterback moving into the pocket, a basketball player resetting a defensive position, or a tennis player retreating from the net to the baseline.

The backpedal is often transitional as well, such as when a football player runs back a few yards to catch a kickoff and then takes it the other way for a touchdown. It shows up when a soccer goalkeeper gets into position on the goal line to thwart a long-range shot and then leaps into the air to push it over the crossbar.

These examples show why it is an essential part of the movement prescription for this stage between rehab and performance.

From a biomechanical standpoint, backpedaling requires knee flexion and extension and hip flexion for leg turnover, and shoulder flexion and extension to swing the arms.

Perhaps the biggest requirement many athletes are missing is the ankle dorsiflexion needed to generate speed from backward steps that begin from an athletic stance.

If athletes are lacking this range of motion, they will overload the soleus and gastrocnemius and sometimes tilt forward to compensate. This is why it is important to pair backpedaling drills with mobility exercises that improve ankle dorsiflexion and reduce excess stiffness in the calves and higher up the posterior chain in the hamstrings and glutes, which also help manage the eccentric component of backpedaling.

## Backpedaling Drill

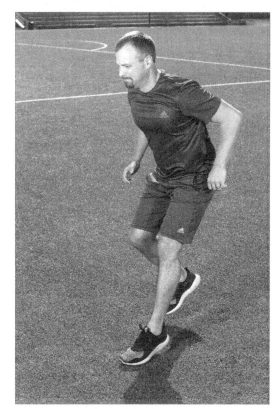

**Photo 10.13—Backpedaling**

*Phase two: As long as there are no apparent issues in phase one, keep increasing the speed of the backpedaling.*

*At the same time, position the athlete lower and lower until starting from the same athletic stance used in the sport.*

*Phase three: Start to add a deceleration element, just like in the deceleration running drill.*

We cover another favorite backpedaling drill on the following page.

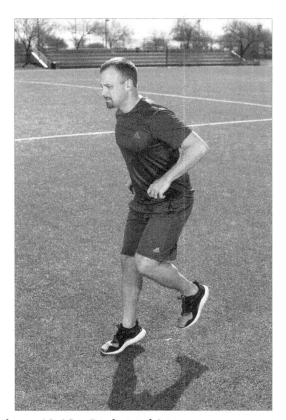

**Photo 10.12—Backward Jog**

*Phase one: With backpedaling, go slowly at first, just as when returning an athlete to running. Begin by having the client walk backward on a treadmill at a very slow speed or on the field and then work up to a backward jog.*

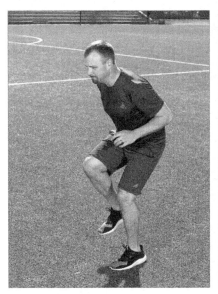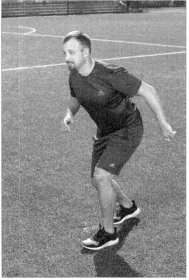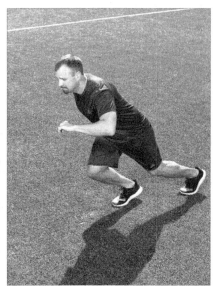

**Photos 10.14a–10.14c—Backpedaling to Forward**

*Phase four: Once the athlete can backpedal at or close to full speed and then decelerate quickly, add in a hard stop followed by sprinting forward for a few yards.*

*Phase five: This step is the same as phase four, but in the transition, have the athlete run left or right after the backpedaling.*

*Phase six: Replace the direction change in the transition with a vertical jump.*

## MULTI-DIRECTIONAL MOVEMENT

The concept of an athletic base is the foundation of all multi-directional movement.

All lateral and rotational movements must originate from an organized, stable, and athletic position if they are to be powerful and sustainable. It is from such a stance that we teach athletes the fundamental concepts of multi-directional movement in a controlled situation.

The following movement progressions form a vital part of the fundamental-advancement stage of rehab.

*Athletic base*

*Shuffle*

*Change of direction*

*Crossover*

*Drop step*

*Open step*

### Athletic Base

The athletic base simply means creating a foundation of multi-directional movement applicable in sports and daily life. If you have an athlete who lacks the ability to get into or hold a solid base position, you cannot work on multi-directional movement. That is why it is the first thing we teach athletes in preparation for agility work.

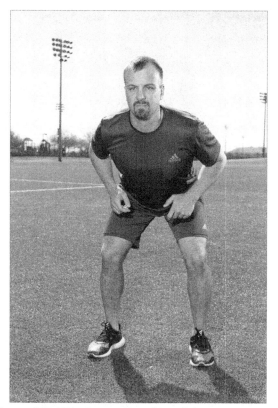

**Photo 10.15—Base, Good Position**

*In an athletic base, the hips are inside the knees, and the knees are inside the feet.*

*The knees are not internally rotated, but are supported by the active hip abductors and external rotators.*

*The feet have a wide base of support and the center of gravity is low for possible movement in any direction.*

Getting into a stable base requires the athlete to stand upright, with feet wider than shoulder width apart. The knees are inside the feet and the pelvis inside the knees, basically forming an "A" position with the lower extremities.

Next, maintaining this foot position, they lower the center of gravity by squatting down. The feet are "screwed into the ground"—the idea is the left foot screws counterclockwise and right foot clockwise—ensuring the hips are active to keep the femurs in an externally rotated position.

If the musculature of the hips, specifically the posterior glute med, are not activated, femoral internal rotation and valgus knees will occur—one or both knees will cave in, placing the knees in a high-risk position.

Upper-body positioning must also be considered, with the chest up, head neutral, and abdominals engaged. The weight is equally distributed between both legs.

The photos on the next page show examples of poor athletic base positions.

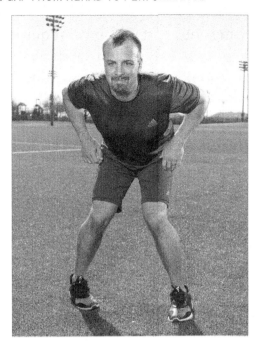 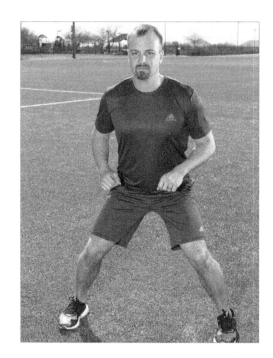

**Photos 10.16a and 10.16b—Base, Poor Position**

*In this position, the athlete does not have as good of a base of support; the knees are in a position of unsupported genuvalgus, and the center of gravity is not low, making movement in any direction more difficult.*

## Shuffle

Once athletes have shown they can form and sustain a stable athletic base, you can begin to get them moving. The shuffle is the first athletic movement to teach out of the base position, as it is so elemental in sports.

Shuffling requires the athletes to maintain the base position as they move right or left. The feet need to stay in the wide stance they started in, as neutral as possible. The hips need to remain active to maintain neutral femurs and well-positioned knees.

The focus in the shuffle is on the athletes pushing off the left leg in order to move to the right, and vice versa. This is in contrast to pulling themselves with the right leg in order to move right.

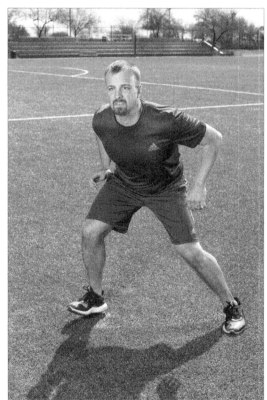

**Photo 10.18—Shuffle, Poorly with Sliding, Foot Externally Rotated**

*In this position, the athlete is pulling forward with the front foot. Note the externally rotated toes, knee, and hip.*

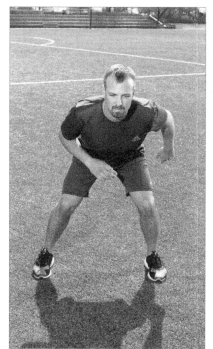 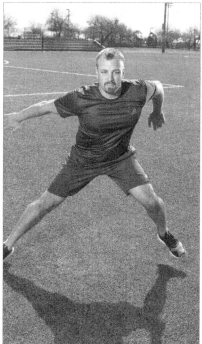 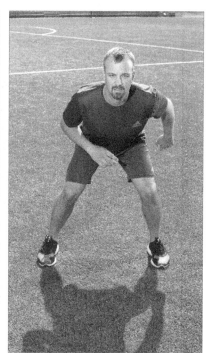

**Photos 10.17a–10.17c—Shuffle**

*From a good athletic base, the athlete pushes in one direction—the movement is driven by the back leg.*

*For example, if the athlete is shuffling to the right, the left leg is driving and pushing the body toward the left by driving the foot into the ground, creating extension in the back leg to push the person in the direction of desired movement.*

*The front leg remains in a neutral position with the toes pointing forward. The front leg does not externally rotate, which would cause the athlete to pull toward the direction of desired movement.*

*The movement is driven by the back leg pushing and extending, not by the front leg pulling and flexing.*

Think about what you would do if your car broke down and you needed to get it to the corner gas station.

Would you push it to the corner, or would you pull it to the corner? You would push.

In this same fashion, teach your athletes to push themselves in the direction they want to go, versus pulling that way.

Once this general motor pattern is established, you can begin to vary speeds and load, adding assistance or resistance depending on the physiological demand you are trying to facilitate.

## Change of Direction

Once the client can independently shuffle in both directions, start to work on change of direction, which is a combination of shuffling both left and right.

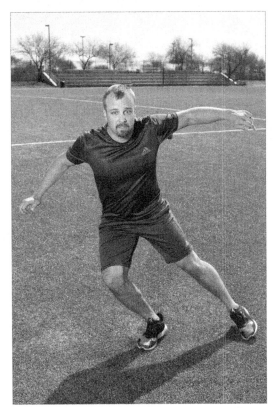

**Photo 10.19—Change of Direction Drill**

*This movement is a progression of the shuffle, asking the athlete to switch directions mid movement. This requires a quick transition for the back leg to become the front leg and vice versa. The quick change of direction requires the athlete to shift the focus of each leg at an instant's notice.*

*The athlete should not have a change in the center of gravity; this is a simple change in direction of movement, keeping all the components of the shuffle during this transition.*

First, have them shuffle right, then switch directions and shuffle back to the left without stopping or pausing. The stance, hip, and chest positions should all generally remain the same when changing direction, noting that lateral trunk movement will alter to shift from right to left, or vice versa. Again, you can add speed, assistance, or resistance as the motor program is ingrained.

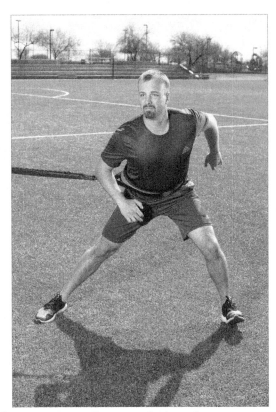

**Photo 10.20—Change of Direction with a Bungee**

*Adding a bungee to one side of the change-of-direction movement causes an assistance in movement in one direction, then a resistance of movement in another.*

*This addition of assistance and resistance to athletic movement can mimic forces an athlete may encounter once back on the field.*

## Crossover

The crossover is a transitional movement that allows athletes to go from a forward-facing position to a complete 90-degree turn.

It is a transitional motion that enables them to combine multi-directional and linear movement.

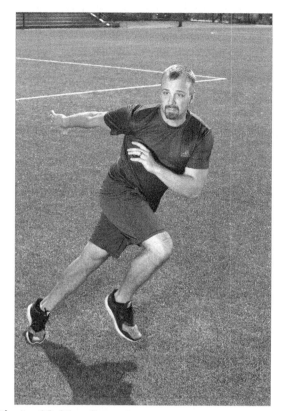

**Photo 10.21—Crossover**

*A crossover maneuver requires the athlete to change direction with a 90-degree ankle, meaning that the athlete will go from an athletic base to an acceleration movement, taking the back leg up and over the front leg.*

*For example, if the athlete is in an athletic base and needs to accelerate to the left, the right leg must quickly and efficiently come in front of the left leg, with the right patella pointing toward the desired direction of movement. The right leg then needs to be able to drive down and back in an acceleration movement to transition from a lateral base into a linear movement.*

Say a football player is facing forward to watch what an opponent is doing, and then decides in an instant to go left for several steps. To do this quickly, the player will cross the right leg in

front of the left to then drive the right leg down and back to initiate acceleration. Athletes also need the capability to reverse this movement sequence to move to the right.

From a bridging-the-gap standpoint, an athlete must be able to attain a stable athletic base, have enough trunk stability to maintain this and have sufficient hip mobility to cross over. We typically use the wall to break this pattern into a progression.

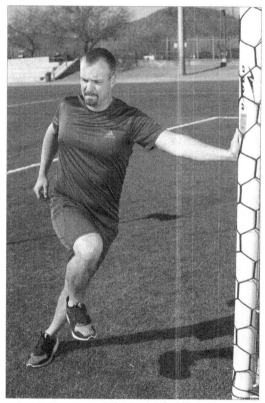

**Photo 10.22—Crossover on a Wall**

*This drill allows us to break down the complexity of the crossover by supporting the athlete on a wall. The task is to take the outside leg toward the wall. The patella of the outside leg needs to point toward the wall as the athlete works on the intricacies of altering the center of gravity and leg position to go from one leg to the other.*

Once the athlete understands the general motor program, we can progress these drills, adding speed, resistance, or assistance, and eventually combine it with other movements to increase the complexity of the drill.

## Drop Step

The drop step allows athletes to go from facing forward to facing in the opposite direction, rotating 180 degrees from the start position.

To do this, they must be able to separate the hips from the pelvis—the femoral acetabular movement on the drop-stepping leg and acetabular femoral movement on the stance leg. Athletes must have good hip mobility, pelvic mobility, and trunk stability to perform the drop step well.

Begin this drill in a standing position to focus on hip and pelvis dissociation, using a wall for stance support if needed.

Once you have established a pain-free movement pattern, move the athlete from the wall to perform a freestanding drop step in both directions.

When your client has demonstrated this ability, start introducing other variables to make it more challenging.

You can also add other previously learned movements to increase the complexity of the movement.

The following are some of my favorite drop step drills.

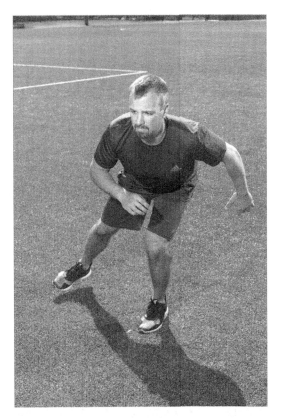 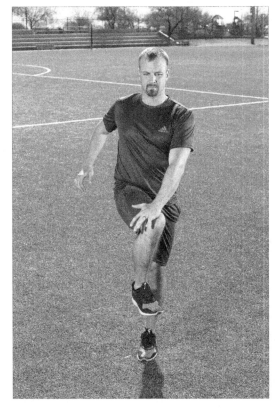

**Photos 10.23a–10.23b—Crossover Exercise, Knee to Hand**

*In the absence of a wall, the hand of the athlete can be used as a target for the knee to hit.*

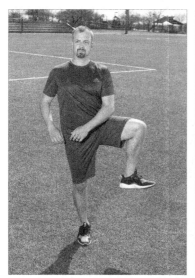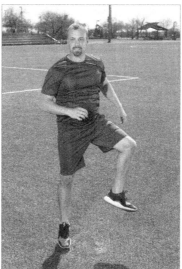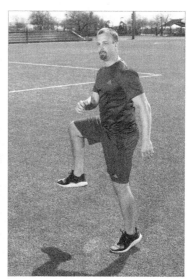

**Photos 10.24a–10.24c—Drop Step Movement**

*The full drop step movement requires the torso to be forward facing, while one leg lifts up into flexion and external rotation. Eventually, the pelvis and then the torso follows, and the lifted leg drives back down into the ground for an acceleration movement. This move is used when an athlete needs to turn 180 degrees.*

*The dissociation of the hip from the pelvis can be practiced next to a wall, using the hand for support as shown in Photo 10.25. This exercise progression allows the athlete to perform the drop step movement away from the stability of the wall in a slow, controlled fashion. Eventually, the drop step can be performed as a skip at a much faster pace.*

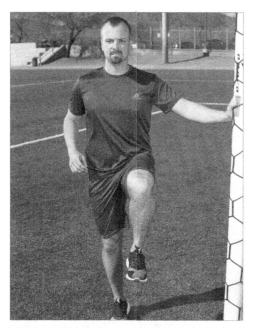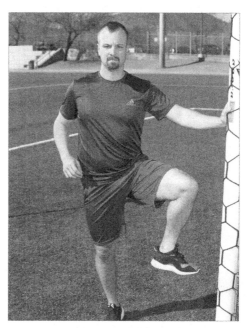

**Photos 10.25a and 10.25b—Wall Dissociation**

*A wall can be utilized to stabilize the torso and upper body while practicing hip and pelvis dissociation in a slow and controlled manner.*

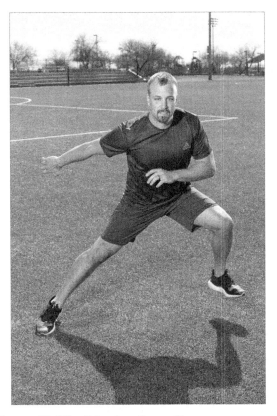

**Photo 10.26—Moving Drop Step**

*This drill has the athlete perform the drop step movement away from the stability of the wall in a slow, controlled fashion.*

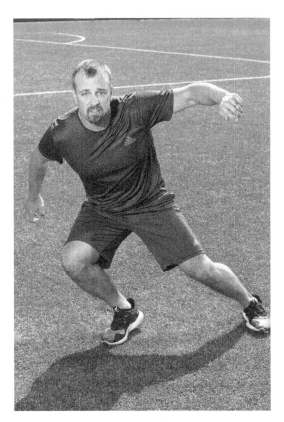

**Photo 10.27—Drop Step Skip**

*Here we add an element of speed to the movement.*

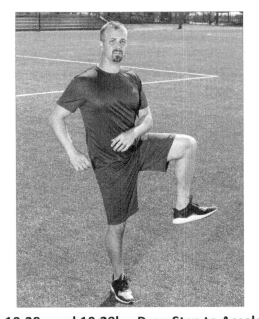

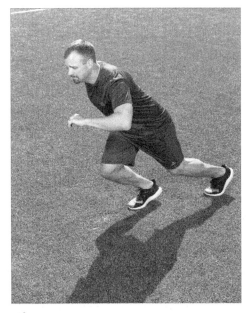

**Photos 10.28a and 10.28b—Drop Step to Acceleration**

*This drill brings complexity to the movement, combining two fundamental movement skills.*

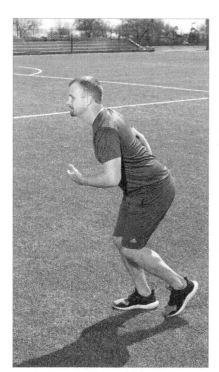 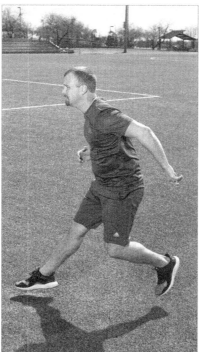 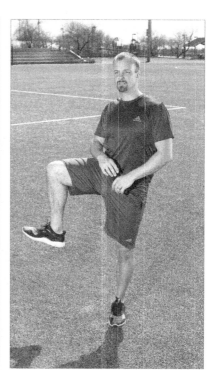

**Photos 10.29a–10.29c—Backpedal to Drop Step**

*The backpedal brings additional complexity to the movement, combining two different fundamental movement skills.*

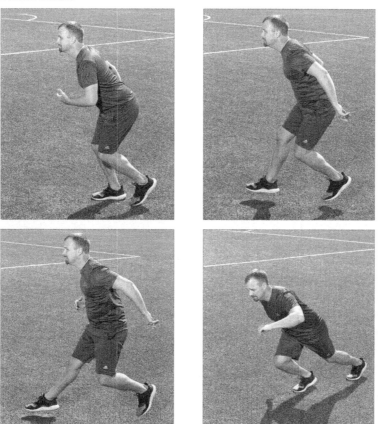

**Photos 10.30a–10.30d—Backpedal to Drop Step to Acceleration**

*Adding greater complexity to the movement, we combine three fundamental movement skills together.*

## Open Step

The crossover and drop steps are not the only common footwork techniques frequently employed in sports.

During Lee Taft's presentation on speed mechanics at the Perform Better Functional Training Summit in 2017, he suggested that the crossover step is probably used less often than we think. He thinks the more simple open step is used often and puts the athletes in a better position to create power in acceleration when transitioning a movement.

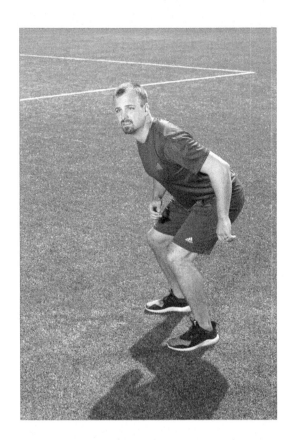

In softball, if a batter is on first base preparing to take the risk of going for second, there are two options. The first is to shuffle a bit and then do a crossover before sprinting.

However, this does not always happen. Some players opt for a second choice, which requires less coordination, but can be initiated more quickly. Instead of crossing the feet over, the player will simply pivot the lead foot, opening the pelvis toward second base, and bring the back leg up into a hip-flexed position to begin acceleration from this position.

We dubbed this "the open step."

**Photos 10.31a and 10.31b—Open Step**

*This is a shift of the pelvis to change direction 90 degrees. The athlete goes from a position of athletic base to acceleration simply by opening up the pelvis in the direction of the desired movement, driving into acceleration from there.*

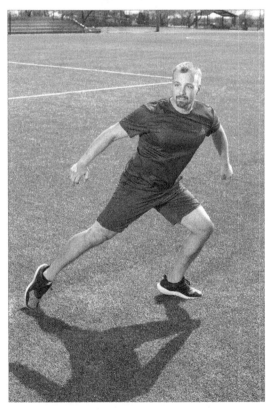

It is worth putting your athletes through a drill that replicates the second option, particularly if you discover it is preferred to the crossover when playing the sport. It is also a good strategy when dealing with an athlete coming back from a labral tear in the hip or an impingement in the lumbar-pelvic region.

## JUMPING AND LANDING

The landing component of jumping is usually just as overlooked as the back-pedaling aspect of running. This comes back to acceleration versus deceleration. We spend a lot of time getting our athletes to jump as high, far, and fast as possible, but devote little to helping them decelerate in a controlled manner so they can absorb the forces created during takeoff. We need to help them with landing safely.

A multi-sport study by Cory Toth found that 60 percent of jump-related injuries are caused by landing improperly.[253] Some studies suggest that landings following a forward jump carry a higher risk than the up-and-down motion of drop jumps, possibly due to explosive movement in multiple directions.[254]

If you throw an apple in the air, it does not splatter on the way up—it smashes when comes down and hits the floor. It is the same with the body's soft tissues. It is possible to sustain an injury when leaping up, but it is far more common to get hurt when we plant our feet back on the ground.

Alignment is one of the main contributing factors in landing-related injuries.

If the joints of the hip, knee, and ankle are centrated and well aligned, they can transmit and absorb great forces without issue. However, when misaligned, we get off-axis shearing that can either cause damage in a single incident or build up to become an injury over time.[255]

Jump studies show that one of the commonalities among young women who tear an ACL is valgus knee, with one or both knees caving inward.[256] This puts an unusually high load on the anterior cruciate ligaments, as well as creating compromises at the hip.

This issue may not begin at the knee, but at the foot and ankle. If the ankle collapses inward when the foot plants and the ankle rolls toward the midline, the knee will follow.

People also get knee issues if the feet are ducked out or pigeoned in. If we are to help people better manage deceleration in landing, we first need to teach better positioning and alignment—literally from the ground up.

### Landing Drills

When we are helping bring an athlete back from injury, jumping and landing are potentially the most hazardous activities due to the high power generation involved. This is why we need to work on alignment of the lower extremities and ensure the person has a solid lumbar-pelvic relationship.

The following is a drill to work on this. You can use a mirror at first for visual cueing and then remove it to help the athlete rely on proprioception.

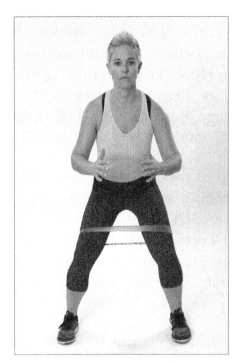 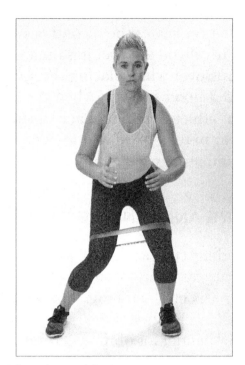

**Photos 10.32a–10.32b—External Rotation with Mini-band in Athletic Base**

*Wrap a stretching or mobility band around the distal femur. Maintain tension on the band while in an athletic base. Allow one hip to internally rotate and then externally rotate against resistance. Repeat on both legs. The athlete should feel this working the posterior hip musculature (gluteal area).*

Make sure the knee is tracking over the second toe and the foot is neutral. Get the athlete to fire the glute medius by squeezing the butt and "screwing" the foot into the ground. This should create a little tension in the band at the distal femur. Reiterate that this is the takeoff and landing position.

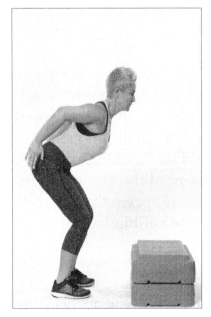 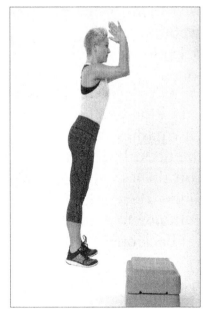 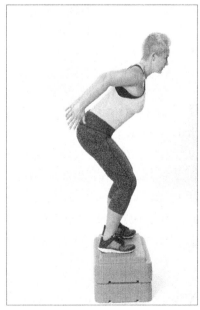

**Photos 10.33a–10.33c—Jump Up to a Box**

*Get the athlete to jump onto a 12-inch box and then step down.*

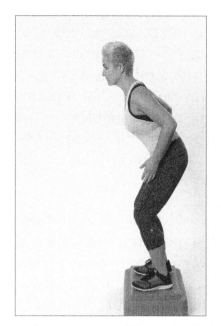 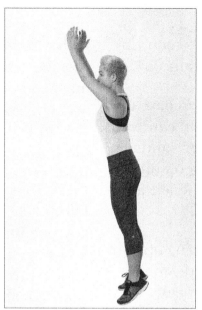 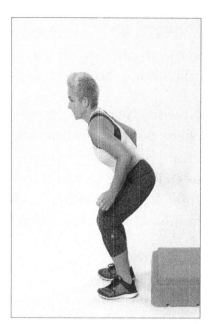

**Photos 10.34a–10.34c—Jump Down to the Floor**

*If the athlete is still displaying correct mechanics and alignment, the next step is to drop down and land from the 12-inch box.*

Stepping down is the key with the drill show in Photos 10.33a—10.33c. At this point, we are simply having the athlete jump up to something. We will work on landing separately.

If the 12-inch box jump is successful, increase the box height to 18 inches.

In this activity, the athlete begins the movement from the top of the box. Have the person simply step up—this is not a jump up to the top of the box. Focus only on the landing portion of the movement.

When you see a consistent, confident landing, repeat with a taller box.

Next, have the athlete jump up onto a box, pause, reposition if needed, and then jump back down. This makes the athlete produce force, dissipate it, and then produce it again, similar to the action of sports, but giving a bit of pause

in the middle to make any adjustments needed before performing the landing portion of the activity.

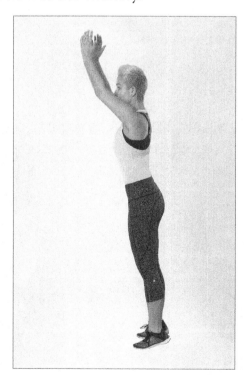

**Photo 10.35—Jump in the Air, No Box**
*Now remove the box to jump into the air and land.*

The drill shown on the previous page in Photo 10.35 removes the pause we allowed on top of the box, requiring adjustments to be made mid-air.

Now try switching directions to have the client do forward bounds. You can program two-footed takeoffs and landings to start, then switch to taking off on the right leg and landing with the left and, finally, reversing the sequence.

Some athletes who are fine going up and down will struggle going side to side, particularly those coming back from an ankle injury that created instability. Make sure they are paying attention to landing softly on a flat foot. The feet are neutral during takeoff and landing, and the ankle, knee, and hip should be in alignment each time.

From here, you have a plethora of options, such as integrating a 90-degree turn mid-jump, a 180-degree turn, moving anterior-lateral at a 45-degree angle, or lateral bounds. The options are endless and are dependent upon the athlete's sport, position and possible movements encountered during the return to play.

Ultimately, an athlete needs to go from any one of these positions to another at a specific time. We need to progress the athlete through an acceleration progression, an absolute speed progression, a deceleration program, multi-directional movement drills, jumping exercises, and landing education and activities.

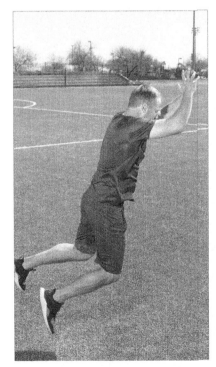 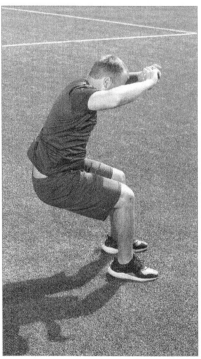 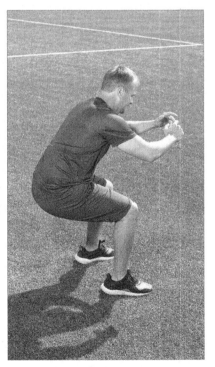

**Photos 10.36a–10.36c—Horizontal Jumps, Two Feet to Two Feet**
*The athlete begins with two feet on the ground and jumps for distance—not height—landing with both feet on the ground.*

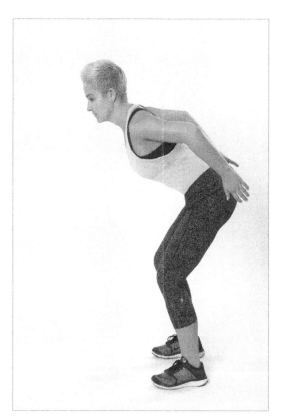 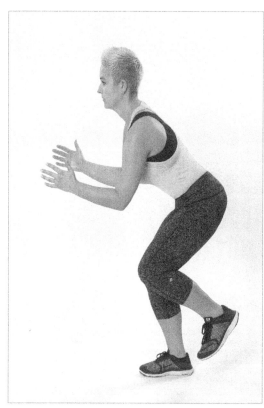

**Photos 10.37a–10.37b—Horizontal Jumps, Two Feet to One Foot**

*The athlete begins on two feet and jumps for distance, landing on one foot.*

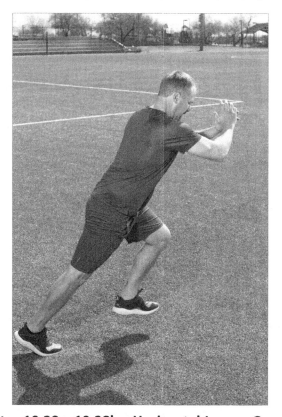 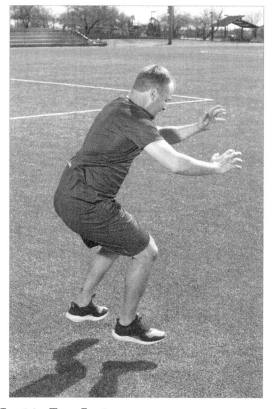

**Photos 10.38a–10.38b—Horizontal Jumps, One Foot to Two Feet**

*This time, the athlete begins with one foot on the ground and jumps for distance, landing with two feet on the ground.*

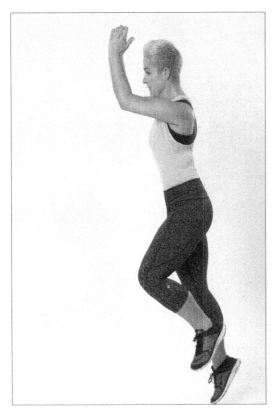 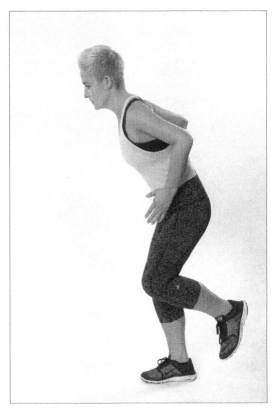

**Photos 10.39a and 10.39b—Horizontal Jumps, One Foot to One Foot**
*The athlete begins on one foot and jumps for distance, landing on one foot.*

Once an athlete has each of these movements down, we combine them. For example, an athlete running down the field will go from acceleration to absolute speed, then decelerate and jump up, then land.

Combining linear and multidirectional movements with jumping and landing are the final athletic movement combinations that need to be checked off before an athlete returns to sport specific movements.

## CLINICAL PEARL
### Fundamental athletic movement patterns you need to understand

- Acceleration
- Absolute speed
- Deceleration
- Athletic base
- Shuffle
- Change of direction
- Drop step
- Crossover
- Open step

## POWER DEVELOPMENT—PLYOMETRICS

The concept of plyometrics is a scary one for anyone coming from the rehab side of our professions. Visions of four-foot box and depth jumps come to mind, creating anxiety for every rehab specialist. However, in the bridging-the-gap continuum, we need to abandon YouTube-worthy feats and return to the true definition of plyometrics, which is the use of the stretch-shorten cycle to produce an explosive movement.

The stretch-shorten cycle involves an eccentric contraction, immediately followed by a concentric contraction. The body uses the stored elastic energy from the eccentric movement to create power in the concentric phase of contraction. This results in an increase in force produced over a short period of time.[257]

For example, when you squat down to jump up, you stretch the quad and glutes. Then your body uses this rubber band–like effect to spring you in the air. It is the difference between throwing a rubber band, and loading it up and letting go, producing much more distance with technically less energy.

Once we understand and respect that definition of the stretch–shorten cycle, almost any athletic movement is plyometric.

Depth jumps are just one form of plyometric work, and do not necessarily need to be used in training, particularly with an athlete coming back from an injury caused by an explosive movement, such as an Achilles tendon tear.

The introduction and progression of plyometric movement is key in bridging the gap from rehab to performance. We began this type of motion when training the components of linear and multi-directional movement.

Understanding plyometrics requires some basic definitions, including:

### Ground reaction force
This is an example of Newton's Law of Reaction—the force is equal in magnitude and opposite in direction to the force the body exerts on the surface through the foot or other body part.

### Pillar strength
Pillar strength refers to static and dynamic stabilization strength through the hips, core, and shoulders.

### Kinetic linking
Kinetic linking is how we transfer energy from one segment to the next.

### Counter movement
Counter movement is the concentric phase of a jump, hop, throw, or other similar movement.

### Center of mass
This is the central point where a body's entire quantity of matter is considered to be concentrated.

### Eccentric
Eccentric action is muscle contraction during which tension is developed while a muscle is lengthening.

### Concentric

Concentric action is the opposite of eccentric—it is muscle contraction where tension is developed while a muscle is shortening.

### Isometric

Isometric contraction is action during which tension is developed while muscle is maintaining constant length.

### Amortization

Amortization is the time from the onset of the eccentric contraction to the onset of concentric contraction.

### Coupling time

Coupling time is the time from the end of the eccentric contraction to the beginning of concentric contraction.

### Jump

Jumping drills involve ground contact with two feet.

### Hop

Hopping is a jumping drill involving ground contact with one foot.

### Bound

Bounding is a jumping drill involving ground contact alternating between feet.

There are different amplitudes of plyometrics we can use in training to:

- *be safe when introducing this concept to someone who has been injured*
- *refine movement to eventually become efficient in the transfer of force for power*
- *improve muscle activation to reduce the chance of future injury*

We can use small or large amplitudes of movement to teach what will ultimately be the optimal amplitude for repeated power production during athletic movement.[258]

These varying plyometric amplitudes are rapid response, long response, very-long response, and short response. See Figure 10.1 on the following page for a graphic depiction.

## Rapid Response

A rapid-response movement is a very low amplitude movement that will produce minimal additional joint stress on the body—think of an agility ladder or other quick-feet work. With this activity, we reintroduce the concept of being elastic versus being heavy footed.

Most rehabilitating athletes have had to be slow and controlled in their movements until this stage in the bridging-the-gap continuum, and this concept of being light and fast is something we need to reintroduce.

When performing a rapid-response drill, we are more concerned about speed than we are about amplitude. The low amplitude will protect the joints; however, this is where we begin to reintroduce the neuromuscular action of quick movements.

## Long Response

Next, we can progress to long-response exercises, where athletes repeat the movement within the same set. The amplitude is a bit larger and they have time to think about what they are doing, the body position, and how they are moving.

For this reason, the time the athlete spends on the ground is increased. A squat jump is a good example of a long-response plyometric.

## Very-Long Response

Very long–response plyometrics are those in which the athlete spends more time on the ground between repetitions, but creates a greater amount of force with each rep.

Maximum vertical leaps or broad jumps are good examples of these drills. We use some long and very-long variations to increase the eccentric load to create greater concentric force. You can also apply resistance by having the athlete use a mobility band or an implement like a barbell or a medicine ball.[259]

During very long–response training, we remove the absorption or eccentric portion of the movement, therefore, by definition, very long–response exercises are not plyometric exercises.

However, the athlete will use the isometric and concentric portion of the movement and eliminate the eccentric action in order to break the movement down, giving the athlete fewer things to focus on.

Very long–response drills can be used to support plyometric training.

## Short Response

Finally, we can focus on short responses, or what would be considered the actual repetitive-movement, stereotypical plyometric exercise.

The rapid-response, long-response and very long–response exercises all build upon or break down different components of a plyometric activity until the athlete finally attempts to put it into a full, short response, typical plyometric movement. These exercises center on single-repetition movements, such as six or eight sets of one.

Once we move to rapid-response exercises, there is no time for thinking. The athletes have to perform several movements in one set and reflexively do the movements, trusting that they are putting everything together well.

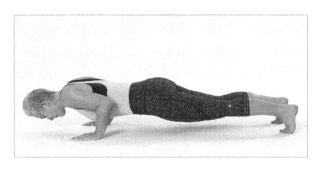

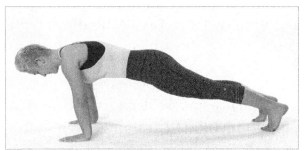

**Photos 10.40a–10.40b—Upper-Extremity Progression of Plyometrics**

*Any movement can be turned into a plyometric activity, whether it is at the upper or lower extremity. Dropping into a plank and then pushing into a pushup position where the hands are off the ground will utilize the stretch–shorten cycle to create power in the upper extremity.*

*Maintaining great trunk stability and positioning will be keys for any upper-extremity plyometric.*

*Keep in mind this is one example—medicine ball activities can also be plyometric for the upper extremity.*

## NON-COUNTER, COUNTER, DOUBLE-CONTACT, AND CONTINUOUS MOVEMENTS

We can use different techniques to teach an athlete how to perform plyometrics in an athletic setting, gradually building on each drill until the client is finally doing a true plyometric exercise.

The main variations we employ are described as non-counter movement, counter movement, double-contact, and continuous movement.

## Non-Counter Movement

Non-counter movements (NCMs) are when we use what we want to be a plyometric exercise, but remove the eccentric portion. We employ NCMs during long or very-long response activities as previously described.

It is arguable that what remains is no longer a plyometric, but NCMs are valuable for teaching movement principles. During an NCM, the athlete starts with the isometric portion of the movement and then performs the concentric portion.

Take, for example, a squat jump: Beginning at the bottom of a squat position, the person simply jumps up. The athlete then returns to the isometric portion of the movement—the bottom portion of the squat jump—and repeats the motion.

## Counter Movement

Next, we introduce the counter movement. This progression reinserts the eccentric portion of the activity. Going back to the example of a squat jump, the athlete would begin standing, drop down, and then jump up one time. The person would then reset and repeat.

Studies have shown that adding a counter movement into the jump-and-land sequence can create more muscular

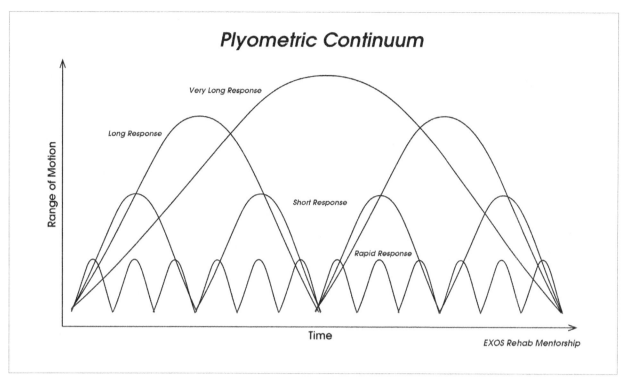

**Figure 10.1—Plyometric Continuum**

*Short-response activities are what most people consider plyometric exercises. However, rapid-response, long-response and very long–response movements can be used to support, teach, and improve the short-response plyometric movement.*

*Rapid response movements teach athletes how to be fast on their feet. These drills are low in amplitude and high in frequency.*

*A very long–response movement has a high amplitude and is done for a single repetition. It removes the eccentric portion of the exercise, which means this drill is not a plyometric exercise; however, it can be used to teach the isometric and concentric portion of the plyometric movement.*

*Long-response movements have a high amplitude and low frequency and use the eccentric portion of the movement. And finally, the athlete is able to express the movement in an optimal amplitude and optimal frequency for power production.*

contraction and also takes advantage of the energy created by tendon elasticity.[260] This is plyometric activity.

## Double-Contact Movement

When using a double-contact movement, we begin to teach repetition within the activity, and in doing so, we start reinforcing the movement pattern.

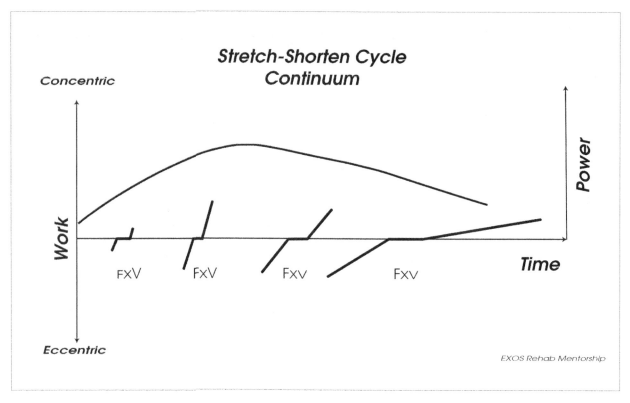

**Figure 10.2—Stretch-Shorten Cycle Continuum**

*This graph shows what we ultimately want to accomplish with plyometric training. In rapid-response movements, there is very little work being done as the movements are low amplitude and high frequency.*

*There is no huge concentric or eccentric demand. In very long–response—the right side of graph–there is a lot of work being done, with very little power being produced.*

*The short response, the second line in the graph, depicts the sweet spot, the place where minimal amount of work is being done by the athlete, yet the greatest power is being created.*

*This type of movement gives us the biggest return on our investment. The return is power production—our investment is the amount of work being done.*

Athletes do not have to fully reuse the energy created during a plyometric. We allow a double-foot contact to reset their posture and think about alignment.

Using our squat jump example, we start the athletes in standing, then drop down, and jump up. Next, the athletes return to the bottom portion of the squat, giving a slight, small-amplitude extra jump at the bottom before jumping up again.

This extra contact at the isometric portion of the movement provides an additional instant of thought during this conscious portion of developing a motor program.

## Continuous Movement Pattern

Finally, you might tell the athletes to perform a continuous movement pattern, in which they would repeatedly jump up and down using the stored energy from the eccentric portion of the movement to create power in the concentric phase.

This is when you will see the true expression of a plyometric.

## TOOLS FOR PLYOMETRIC TRAINING

The beauty of plyometric training is that we can do the drills anywhere, with minimal equipment. Simply using bodyweight activities and manipulating the stretch-shorten cycle is all that is needed to institute a plyometric program.

Of course, tools can enhance our programming. Things like kettlebells, med balls, and Olympic lifting can all enhance our expression of plyometric training and can be used when appropriate, based on your instructing ability and the athletes' experience level.

Olympic lifting is such an unbelievable tool for power development, but you need to have the foundational movements down and practice coaching for a long time to do it well.[261]

Going into the full scale of this training is beyond the scope of this book, but there are great resources in Appendix Nine for your further study if this not already in your toolbox.

## PLYOMETRIC TRAINING AND ITS RELATIONSHIP TO FASCIA

Plyometric training is often thought of and referred to as training muscles as described above. However, new research regarding fascial training has brought us full circle to see plyometrics in a new light.

Muscle strength and the stretch-shorten cycle as it relates to muscle does not give us the full picture of training. We have to consider fascial strengthening since it is a force transmitter, as previously discussed.

Multi-directional, multi-angular movement is key to fascial training. Small movements in the muscle can create stored energy in the tendon, collagen, and fascia. Storage capacity of connective tissue is important when it comes to reaping the kinetic energy benefits of this tissue.

Think of a kangaroo. Is the kangaroo stronger or more powerful than other animals that it can hop incredible distances? Or does the kangaroo's connective tissue have incredible ability to store and release energy thanks to a preparatory countermovement? We are finding it is the latter.[262]

These findings do not necessarily change the fact that we should use plyometric training in our programming, but further research may clarify why we are using plyometric training and how it works.

## SUMMARY

Returning an athlete to fundamental linear and multi-directional movement is necessary to bridge the gap from rehab to performance. You must be able to understand these movement patterns and be able to break them down based on the athlete's needs to work in this space.

Health care professionals should seek the advice of a strength coach to better understand these movements and the nuances between acceleration and absolute speed, or a shuffle versus a crossover movement.

Strength and conditioning coaches should seek the advice of a health care professional to safely implement and manipulate the training variables for a person who is returning from injury. This is an area where your referral network is vital.

Using the foundations of strength, recovering athletes should be able to move within these foundational athletic patterns at varying loads and speeds in preparation for their sport-specific movement patterns.

# CHAPTER ELEVEN
## THE FINAL PHASE—
## ADVANCED PERFORMANCE

In the previous chapter, we looked at some of the fundamental performance considerations that apply to helping an athlete prepare to return to competition. As we move into the final phase of the rehab continuum, it is time to get more specific.

All our clients have unique requirements for their sports. The games they play have unique demands on multiple bodily systems—including cardiovascular, structural-anatomical, and energy substrate—due to the nature of each game.

There are sport-specific and position-specific skills and motor patterns your clients will need to hone before they again start playing their sports.

As you read in the Pain Generator chapter beginning on page 39, pain resulting from injury can not only lead to a player favoring the non-injured side long after acute symptoms fade, but can also alter wiring in the brain areas responsible for movement. This means we have extra skills-based work to do to get our athletes ready to play a sport after injury.[263]

We also need to address the differing needs of the recreational athlete. If your clients sit at a desk all day and play golf on the weekends, they will have different requirements than professional or college athletes. Pros and everyday Joes alike need the universally applicable skills we focused on in the fundamental-advancement phases we just covered, but now that we are moving into the advanced performance stage, we need to get client-specific.

What fine-tune tweaking does a program need to individualize the final phases of a journey back to full competition? This is what we will discuss in this section.

## TRANSITIONING FROM FUNDAMENTAL TO ADVANCED PERFORMANCE

Although they share fundamental athletic principles, each sport and each position within that sport has different needs from a movement skills perspective. We need to coach each athlete slightly different, and individualize the rehab at the tail end before the client returns to full participation readiness.

Think about acceleration. If you are working with a defensive back or a wide receiver, the player will be on the line of scrimmage in a split stance, a position similar to an offensive or defensive lineman.

The center of gravity will be low, but not as low as someone on the offensive or defensive line. This means the starting point from which they generate starting speed is different.

Contrast this to a baseball player on first base, who is set to run and perhaps slide toward second to steal the base. The starting stance will be entirely different from those of any football player.

In all three positions, we have athletes preparing to move into acceleration. All of them will need to generate speed, as discussed in more detail in the previous chapter. The differences lie in the position from which they will be accelerating.

The wide receiver or defensive back will have a slight split stance and a low center of gravity. The linemen will have a wider split stance and a lower center of gravity. The baseball player will be in an athletic base, moving from a lateral to a forward position with a low center of gravity.

The mechanical needs in applying acceleration will vary, not to mention the endpoint at which they need to either decelerate or change direction.

Even an athletic element like acceleration that seems simple and universal on the surface is anything but simple. Multiply this by all the stances and movement variations for each position, and you can see why it is invaluable to involve dedicated sport-specific skills coaches.

When coaching a variety of athletes, it is important to understand the necessities of their positions on the team and the postures through which they will be moving. Athletic movement is random and unpredictable and an athlete should be prepared to move into and out of every movement archetype into every other one in the sport.

We can use our knowledge of their sports and positions to better prepare them for the specific movements and transitions they will need when returning to competition.

It is not enough to help remove pain and get a motion segment moving. We must also help the athlete efficiently and effectively move the affected area in sequence with the rest of the body and in the context of the motions of every team practice session and game.[264]

## THE IMPORTANCE OF SKILLS COACHES

Whenever possible with your athletes, plan to include a skills coach throughout the rehab process, but especially in this final phase. It is imperative to make sure the client has checked the boxes for every sport-specific requirement.

People ask about my transition when working with different sports, for example in-season baseball to in-season soccer. How different and difficult was it? Parts of the switch were hard and others were not. At the end of the day, a second baseman and a soccer player both need to run. I understand running and know the difference between acceleration and absolute speed.

When I moved from working with baseball players to soccer players, I needed to learn the difference between running around the bases in a defined, repetitive pattern versus zigzagging around moving obstacles that could be anywhere on the soccer pitch with a ball at a player's feet.

I needed expert help to fully grasp those differences and their implications for rehabbing these athletes, particularly in the final stage of the continuum before clearing them to return to active status.[265]

It would not be enough to reach out to other PTs who had worked with athletes in other sports. What I needed was the help of skills coaches who understood every angle of each sport and could teach me the technical nuances of them.

## PREPROGRAMMED VERSUS RANDOM MOVEMENTS

In Chapter Eight, beginning on page 135, we explored some of the fundamental performance elements we need to work on once our athletes have recovered full function.

In this stage of learning or relearning, running, backpedaling, acceleration, deceleration, and the other skills mentioned are preprogrammed. We give the athletes set parameters as we scale each one.

In the example of basic deceleration on page 201, we effectively prescribed all the conditions of the drill: direction of forward movement, effort level at top speed, sprinting distance of 40 yards, and deceleration distance of 20 yards.

Such preprogrammed drills are highly effective in increasing overall physical preparedness and grooving functional and sustainable skills and positions common to all sports. However, as you know, sports games are not controlled environments with predefined criteria.

They are chaotic, with very little predictability and an almost infinite number of variations in each event due to the complex interactions between the ball, teammates, opponents, surface, weather conditions, chance, and many other variables.

Sports games require the performance of more open skills, of which the execution is determined by the unique stimuli in any instant of the game. Open skills are more physically and mentally demanding than closed skills, such as those performed in a controlled environment on the practice field.[266]

We can never fully mirror an actual sports game, with the possible exception of a full-sided, full-contact scrimmage. Even then, we are missing the roar of the crowd and the resultant adrenaline that accompanies playing a sport in front of thousands or tens of thousands of people. This will affect the potential intensity of the scrimmage, and therefore will not replicate game speed.

What we can do—once we have run through fundamental performance exercises—is introduce some of the game's randomness and chaos into our drills, which will help prepare a body and brain for competition.

## IT IS NOT WHAT YOU SAY, IT IS HOW YOU SAY IT

Working with competitive athletes is not just about gaining a greater insight into the technical skills and the movement patterns upon which they are based.

We also may have to learn a new language. If we want to fit in within the new sport we are working with, we have to alter our vocabulary between things like "batting practice" to "training" and "the field" to "the pitch."

Even small differences in how we communicate with coaches and athletes will have an impact on how well we can get our points across. This also affects how well we absorb their input, which will better separate sport-specific training from general performance training.

Understanding sport terminology helps us communicate with the players, and it helps us understand what the players are saying.

Early in my days of baseball, a player said he "got jammed at the plate." This means the pitcher threw inside and the batter was unable to swing the way he wanted. This can result in awkward movements and consequently, often some pain at the wrist or hand.

I had been thinking he jammed his finger, and was trying to look at his finger while he looked at me as if I was crazy. Knowing the language your athletes is using will help you look more intelligent to your athletes, and will help with your assessments based on their subjective reports.

As a specialist, you need to acknowledge that even if you have been using certain terminology for a long time and think you are good at making others understand you, you still need to update your internal dictionary to the words and phrases the head coach, positional coaches, and players prefer.[267]

This helps with clarity of message as it also helps ensure there is no dissonance or conflict between what you are telling your client and what the coaches are saying.

Time is another reason to abandon your technical terms in favor of the sport's everyday usage. You only have a limited amount of time to spend with each person and if you spend much of it trying to unravel words, you are not going to have time to put your ideas into action.

## USING VISUAL, AUDIBLE, AND TACTILE CUES

During a sports game, cueing is one of the triggers for a player to access the appropriate movement pattern. The three most common cue types are:

*Visual*—This is something the player sees, such as a hand signal on the line of scrimmage or a forward pointing to the rim to get the point guard to throw an alley-oop pass.

*Audible*—An audible is a spoken cue a player hears, such as "screen left" to let a basketball player know a defender is about to get in the way.

Another example is a quarterback's improvised play call...or Seabiscuit turning on the speed when he heard his trainer ring the bell at the race track.

*Tactile*—A tactile cue is a touch-based cue a player feels. This could be a sensation from the ball or an opponent leaning on a soccer player's left side, which causes a spin and dribble away to the right.

As we have already seen, pain and the other aftereffects of injury can play havoc with an athlete's brain and body. Some of these disruptions can be to the senses, which in turn hampers the connection between visual, audible, and tactile feedback coming in via the peripheral nervous system to be processed by the CNS.[268]

Bad input equals bad output when it comes to movement. In order for an injured player to be ready to get back in the game, we need to help improve input quality and enhance the feedback loop between sensation and action.

There are many examples for different sports and positions. You will find one for each cue category below.

## Visual Cue Drill

Think back to that baseball player trying to steal second. When helping get this player back to competition readiness, we might try a drill in which the athlete will stand on a makeshift first base and start shuffling to the side. The player should only turn and sprint to the object you are using for second base when you raise your arm in a certain way, while disregarding any of your other movements.

This type of drill homes in on the visual cues needed to successfully steal a base when base running; it is a visual cue to set off the motor program of stealing a base.

## Audible Cue Drill

When an offensive lineman is in a crouched stance waiting for the play to begin, it is easy to be distracted by the hand movements and chatter of the opposing defensive line, talk among the teammates, and the crowd noise. When an athlete is injured, the ability to process audible cues can be disrupted while focused on the movement execution.

Here again we need to improve the ability to focus on the quarterback's audible play call while disregarding all other stimuli.[269] We may get the player into the stance and then start calling out colors: green, red, yellow, and so on. The player is to remain still until hearing the call of "blue," which is the signal to explode forward off the line as if charging toward a defensive lineman on the opposite side.

## Tactile Cue Drill

One of the best examples of an athlete using a tactile cue in competition is a relay runner waiting to receive the baton from a teammate. This runner will start getting up to speed, but will not turn on the jets until feeling the baton in hand, although sometimes there is also the audible cue of the other runner shouting "Hand!"

You could replicate this drill exactly or have the athlete face away from you and only turn and sprint when feeling your touch on the arm or shoulder.

## ASSISTED VERSUS RESISTED VERSUS COMBINATION MOVEMENTS

As another compare-and-contrast concept of the fundamental movements and skills of Chapter Nine, we need to cover assisted and resisted movements. In that chapter, beginning on page 173, we did not add any variables that encouraged or discouraged movement in any plane of motion.

However, in a team sports game, the athlete does not act in isolation, and contact with other players will either assist or resist the momentum. This can involve impeding or accelerating motion in the preferred direction or forcing the person to either resist or succumb to forces channeled on a different plane.[270]

When a wide receiver is getting ready to leap for a pass, the player has to go from sprinting to leaping up in the air. However, the cornerback has other ideas and leans in with the upper body in an attempt to disrupt the intended action. We could say the wide receiver has to perform the skills of running and jumping as resisted movements.

In sport, we also have situations in which players might be propelled in a

given direction faster than they would be moving under their own steam.

For example in rugby, the players who are lifted up to try to catch the ball in the lineout are assisted by the vertical power applied by their teammates; they are much higher in the air than if they had jumped.

The third type of movement is a combination, in which conflicting forces both assist and resist player motion. Using another rugby example, we have the maul, where a couple of offensive players try to move a teammate onward while defenders bind onto the tackler to try to stop the offensive team from advancing.

Combination movements are often multi-directional and require athletes to manage assistive and resistive forces, as well as their own self-generated movement, and this is through multiple planes of motion.

The collisions involved in recreating such realistic game-like scenarios are the last thing you want to impose on a rehabbing client. Nevertheless, it is possible and even desirable to introduce some external forces that either assist or resist motion or simultaneously do both.

By doing so, you can further challenge the integrity of the athlete's movement patterns and "battle test" in a semi-controlled environment before returning to the field. This alleviates some of the risk that comes with full-contact drills.

Some examples of tools to employ in this area include sleds and bungees. A sled provides the option of resisting motion in two different directions, depending on whether you have the athletes pull it behind them using a harness, push it ahead, or pull it toward them using a strap or rope. You can also create an imbalanced load by weighting one side of the sled with a heavier load than the other side.[271]

You can use bungees to create assisted or resisted loads in partner drills based on the direction you pull and where the athlete is in relation to you. For a greater level of control, you can attach the bungee to a belt or harness for the athlete to wear.

As well as using them to assist or resist forward and backward motion, bungees or resistance bands also provide the opportunity to resist jumping or create side-to-side or off-axis resistance for the athlete to work against. You can use multiple bungees or bands to make a combination of multidirectional resistance and assistance.

## GETTING A TOOL BACK IN AN ATHLETE'S HANDS

It is possible to prepare an athlete for a return to competitive play with isolated drills and movements. However, if you can use a tool of the sport, you will improve readiness by putting that implement back in hand during this advanced performance stage, or even possibly earlier in the continuum. This could be a bat for a baseball player, a racquet for a tennis player, or whatever tool or tools a sport requires your clients to use.[272]

Of course, it is important to get your athletes moving well in the earlier stages of the bridging-the-gap model. Once they have recovered the required range of motion and motor control and you have worked on the fundamental performance components, it is time to start making the drills more realistic and specific to their games of choice. Until then, you have hypothetically got them ready without providing any degree of realism.[273]

This principle does not only apply to those players who wield bats, racquets, and clubs. It is also relevant to anyone who uses a ball. If you are working with rugby, basketball, or football players, you have to get that ball back in their hands, and if it is soccer or they do a lot of kicking in another sport, you need the ball back at their feet.

Often, movement will normalize once the player has the necessary implement in hand or at foot. The recovering athlete most likely has been performing the skill for years, and the motor programs necessary for each sport are well ingrained in the nervous system even though the motor patterns have been disrupted by injury. Often, these inherent movements come back as soon as the athlete has the necessary equipment, enhancing movement quality.

This is why many coaches do not just want their players running around the field, court, or pitch, but instead want them to participate in small-sided games and drills in which they have to move or stop the ball. After all, that is what they have to do during a game or match.

It is the same in the rehab context: A recovering athlete does not regain the confidence of feeling like a player until starting to work with a ball or tool.

Your injured players will start feeling like part of a squad again once they begin dribbling, shooting, or passing after coming out of rehab.

Before that, some will have trouble with the mental aspect of separation from both their teammates and their sport's implements. As soon as they are able to start getting their touch back, they will feel more ready to come back to full practice or games.

Implementing the use of an athlete's sport-specific tool as early as possible in the rehab process is advantageous from a mental aspect as well. It benefits the player to get out of a rehab frame of mind and into a performance mindset, and quite often using a racquet, bat, or tool of choice will help people make this transition.

Physically, mentally, and emotionally, incorporating a sport-specific tool in this advanced stage is imperative, whether or not you used it earlier in the rehab process.

## IMPLEMENTS AND MOVEMENT

Before an athlete returns to practice scenarios such as one-on-one or three-on-three in basketball, you can combine use of the ball or tool with movement-specific exercises similar to those skills a full game requires. You can also use the field of play to make the scenarios even more

appropriate and as similar to the game as possible.

In tennis, for example, once a player can run forward and backward, the runs can be between the baseline and the net. Once able to move laterally with no ill effects, try using a shuffle back and forth along the baseline.

Next, reintroduce a racquet into the picture; this might be a run to the net with the racquet in hand and then backpedal to the baseline. Then, still holding the racquet, ask for a shuffle from side to side across the net and along the baseline.

Even though you have not yet added a ball or a training partner to hit it back, combining back-front and lateral drills with the implement will start firing the motor cortex and other areas of the brain responsible for movement.

As soon as the athlete is comfortable using the tool again, you can add balls from a machine, and soon you can include a hitting partner.

## USING MOVEMENT ANALYSIS

Another thing to consider is a movement analysis to break down a player's complex movement patterns to see how these relate to the specific requirements of the sport and position. The goal is to make it easier to retrain sport-specific motions to advance players along the rehab continuum.

As its name suggests, a movement analysis identifies every common action of a sport, and then breaks each down into start and finish positions and the movements in between.

Let us look back at tennis to provide a couple of examples. A player receiving a serve would typically start in an athletic stance on or just behind the baseline and then move left or right, often using a crossover step to get to the ball.

Next, the player would plant both feet and rotate the trunk to initiate the return. Once the ball comes off the racquet, the player shuffles laterally to again establish a central position for a better reaction to the opponent's next shot.

This could potentially send the athlete sideways or rushing to the net, maybe to hinge at the hips to get to a drop shot or to stop running forward, plant the feet, and extend the racquet sideways to reach a passing shot.

Once we label the action and list the starting and stopping positions and movements, we then assign certain drills that take place during the advanced performance stage.

By the end of the process, we have created a list of events with corresponding movements, positions, and transitions, along with drills both with and without the tool that allow us to layer on complexity and speed as the athlete's rehab progresses.

First, we might start with the more fundamental performance elements of acceleration and deceleration. Then we could move on to sport-specific contexts within certain skills or actions, such as returning a tennis serve.

Using a movement analysis in this way helps us as professionals, and it also helps our athletes. When looking at the big picture, returning to sporting competition can seem daunting and sometimes even an insurmountable challenge.

When breaking down the final stages of the rehab continuum into small, tangible acts, we encourage athletes to focus on each step and be present in the moment.

This helps them concentrate physical and mental efforts on definable, actionable, and achievable goals, rather than worrying about what they cannot yet do and catastrophizing with negative self-talk phrases like, "It is too hard. I am never going to make it back."

If you can get them to home in on and celebrate small victories, they will avoid the negative mindset that can hamper recovery and slow the achievement of the ultimate goal.

## CREATING A MOVEMENT ANALYSIS

To create a movement analysis, you need a great understanding of the sport you are analyzing. If you do not have a great knowledge of the sport, you need to learn from someone who does, including your athlete.

When I first started working at what was then called Athletes' Performance, I worked with some high-level baseball players. I did not yet know very much about the intricacies of the game, hitting mechanics, or throwing mechanics, and I did not try to act like I did.

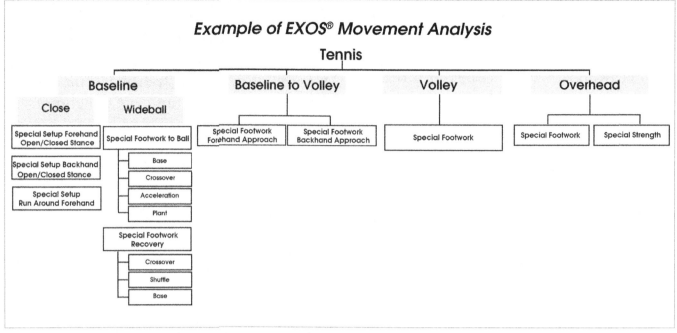

**Figure 11.1—Example of EXOS Movement Analysis**

*When creating a movement analysis, you will list the main movements that need to be performed.*

*Under each general category, all the finer points that create those large categories are also listed. These movements continue to be broken down until you get to the fundamental athletic movement that needs to be performed.*

*Once we identify the building blocks of each major movement that needs to be performed in a sport, we can work on the fundamental movement patterns as described in Chapter Ten, combining them into the larger movement.*

I understood the body and the injuries the clients were dealing with; they presented their knowledge and I presented mine, and we figured things out together. I watched a lot of film with them. We reviewed hitting, throwing, running, and fielding, and then we talked it out.

I asked them to show me the stance, then we viewed film to see if was the same. We watched in slow motion, breaking down every crossover and maneuver the athletes did. We eventually created plans for return to play and executed from there.

My point: Do not try to act like an expert in an area if you are not one. The athletes will always know when you are bluffing or are unsure of what you are saying as you use the wrong language. Talk to experts, do some reading, watch film, and talk with your athletes. These are the first steps to creating a movement analysis.

From there, you should be able to pick out small movements they perform, using the movement categories discussed earlier in this book. What types of linear and multi-directional movements do they perform and how do they need to link these together? We cannot put a sequence together if we cannot perform the parts.

For example, soccer player needs to be able to head the ball. Heading the ball consists of accelerating to get up to speed, possibly transitioning to absolute speed, and then jumping to head the ball. In order for soccer players to run and head the ball, they need acceleration, possibly absolute speed, jumping, and landing.

Returning to performance training, we work on acceleration mechanics, absolute speed mechanics, jumping, and landing techniques on different days until they begin to master each movement component. Once they do, we combine the parts.

We might have them run for a distance of 30 meters to change from acceleration to absolute speed. We might have them perform a task where they run toward a target and then jump up to hit something. Then we introduce more movement variability by adding a moving ball to hit while jumping. The programming combinations are endless.

That is one movement sequence a soccer player may encounter. What are others? What sequences would a different type of athlete utilize? Once you understand the components of athletic movement, you can put these components together to create realistic situations for which a recovering athlete needs to prepare.

To complete a movement analysis, you need to study and break down every movement pattern your athletes might need to perform and the order in which they perform, as in the earlier tennis and soccer examples. You need to decide what activities they execute and categorize them accordingly.

For example, baseball players need to throw, hit, run the bases, and field. Let us take hitting: They start in a hitting stance, swing, and then run to first as fast as possible, make a decision about trying for second…or even third, depending on the hit.

Depending on whether hitters are left or right handed, they will have different steps out of the box that need to transition into acceleration. Certainly, they will have to accelerate through first base, hitting the bag as they go. They may make a decision to round first and head for second, where they need to slide, either head or feet first.

In this movement analysis, we have a stance, transition steps to acceleration, and deceleration. We might have stance, transition steps, acceleration, curve-linear running, and sliding. Each of these elements must be individually addressed and then be put together as a whole.

We would do the same analysis for base running, fielding a position, and throwing scenarios.

Movement analyses creation can seem daunting. However, once they are prepared, you will have a blueprint for all the athletes you work with as they bridge the gap from rehab to performance.

## BRING IN THE EXPERTS

At Athletes' Performance, I was fortunate to work with some of the best in the performance business, including Mark Verstegen, Darryl Eto, Joe Gomes, Luke Richesson, Craig Friedman, Brandon Marcello, and many others.

Yet despite this wealth of experience, we recognized that to create effective rehab plans and tools such as a movement analysis, our knowledge of how the human body works would not be enough.

We also needed the ability to apply the next-level techniques and ideas we were developing to specific sports. We needed the insider smarts that only skills coaches could provide.

For example, when working with soccer players, we needed the insight of coaches who had worked with soccer players at the highest level.

This also went deeper in some sports, in which there are different skill sets of the various positions. In football, we needed input from quarterback, receiver, running back, O-line, and D-line coaches who really knew the sport.

With their help, the movement analysis we created for the athletes was not only research-driven and sound from a sports-science perspective, but also passed practical muster.

This was particularly important in the advanced performance stage, when we had already covered the basic universal athletic competencies and needed to help players hone the skills they would soon showcase on the field of play.

Such an inclusive approach must come from a place of humility. You might consider yourself one of the best in your profession. That is great, but you do not know everything.

We need to constantly remind ourselves that our primary mission is restoring the health of our athletes—this work is about them, not us. Ego and pride and the silos they create get in the way of achieving that objective.

By admitting we do not know everything and committing ourselves to a continual, never-ending learning process throughout our careers, we will better serve our clients. This, in turn, will help us achieve whatever personal aspirations we might have.

When I was working in pro baseball, I was helping rehab a player who was returning from elbow surgery. Before I started working with him on advanced performance drills, I took a literal step back and watched him interact with an experienced pitching coach. Though his background, education, and life experiences varied greatly from my own, both the coach and I had the welfare of the player as our number-one priority.

At one point, we were both trying to say the same thing, but the coach knew the player well and spoke the same language. I began to take notes of how he referred to certain concepts, and worked hard to incorporate those into my subsequent sessions.

Non-verbal communication is crucial in skill development, and I paid close attention to what the coach was trying to show the player without using words.[274] As a result, this pitcher got back in the lineup ahead of schedule and did better than anyone expected in his first games back.

This was only possible because I was willing to avoid pursuing my own agenda, to admit I did not know anywhere near as much as that brilliant coach, and to take his lead in how he communicated with the pitcher.

I learned a similar lesson watching Jurgen Klinsmann coaching the U.S. Soccer men's national team. This was a man who won the World Cup and multiple club trophies as a player and who, as an international coach, led a largely overlooked team to a much better record than expected.

I watched how he talked with the players and observed how he constructed game-like drills. From this learning experience, I was able to tailor our rehab progressions in a much more sport-specific manner.

These lessons do not apply to just baseball and soccer—they work with any kind of skill or positional coach, or a head coach in any sport. Ask questions, test the theories, and grasp the vernacular. Make it clear you respect them and want to pick their brains for the good of their players. Most will be very happy to share what they know and to get involved in the final stages of the rehab process.

Most coaches will also be eager to help the players feel like they are still a part of the team while working the way back to the starting lineup. Coaches often want to assist your efforts to prevent injured players from feeling isolated—an all too common psychological reaction to injury.[275]

## CREATING AND IMPLEMENTING A RETURN-TO-COMPETITION TIMELINE

As an athlete gets over the pain and other acute issues following an injury, recovers full physical function, and begins sport-specific drills, the excitement about the return to play will build rapidly. Recovering athletes are eager to get back with their teammates; the coaches want a full squad to choose from, and the fans and media also get in on the act.[276]

Such enthusiasm can put pressure on you to rush a player back before fully ready in mind and body. You must resist such external pressure, especially if you think of yourself as a people pleaser. Your job is not to keep the fans, media, coaches, or even the players happy. It is above all to take the best possible care of the athlete's health.[277]

To help make sure this happens, you should follow these three simple steps.

> ## CLINICAL PEARL
>
> ### One—Create the return-to-competition plan:
> Create short-term goals to reach the long-term goal.
>
> ### Two—Get everyone on board:
> Communicate with all parties, including the front office, coaching staff, agents, patient, and other medical staff.
>
> ### Three—Stick to the plan:
> Progress or regress the athlete according to progress being made. Do not allow outside forces and pressures to alter your plan for a safe return.

## Create a Return-to-Competition Plan

Working backward from the date you have outlined for a player to return to competitive play, set up milestone dates along the way, such as "Start running by March 22" or "Play in three-on-three drills by May 12."

When creating the plan and setting the timeline, include every specialist involved in athlete care and performance, and make sure your timing and theirs is aligned.

By working backward from the target date, you can give the athlete ample time to gradually increase the intensity, duration, and frequency of the activities.

When an athlete does not hit one of the milestones along the way, you know the return-to-play date is probably going to be pushed back.

Using milestone markers, you will know this as soon as possible, giving everyone time to process the new goal and the delay in return to competition. There will be no surprises as the date approaches, and the athlete is "suddenly" not available to return as planned.

It is important to be open to moving the athlete back along the rehab-to-performance continuum to spend more time at a previous stage if there is a problem of any kind.

This sometimes happens at a point when the athlete is close to returning to the lineup. For example, you require a baseball player to be able to handle two minor league games before rejoining the major league team. If, after the trial games, pain, movement restriction, or some other issue results, that player is not ready to take the final step of return to play.

As an example of how to think this through, say a player needs to return to competition on the 30th. You might decide to prescribe a week of full practice with no restrictions, which means to participate fully in practice on the 23rd.

In order to do that, it will require several days of random movement work and you need to be doing this by the 19th.

Before you implement random movements, you might be working on preprogrammed multi-directional movements for a week—thus, this needs occur by the 12th. There must be a week of linear movement before that, needing to be running at full speed by the 5th.

Keep working backward in this way until you have mapped out the return-to-play program.

## Get Everyone on Board

If the player and coaching staff know what to expect and you keep them informed of progress and setbacks along the way, they will understand your position and plan.

In this stage, it is vital to provide frequent updates to all stakeholders, particularly the head coach and the athlete, along with reasons for whatever decisions you make that affect the timeline.

Make people feel like partners in the process at every stage and things will go smoothly, with fewer objections and less friction.

## Stick to the Plan, Regardless of Outside Forces

Even if you have to say it every day, make it clear that the health and wellbeing of the athlete is the top priority, and that rushing the plan will jeopardize this.

When professional athletes are in a contract year, they are eager to return to play to prove their worth. In this situation, you need to explain that if they come back too soon, they might not have a career at all. You sometimes have to save athletes from themselves.

At certain stages in the season, the head coach will be under even more pressure than usual to win. However, a win-at-all-costs mentality will only jeopardize an injured athlete if you allow this to impact the timeline. You cannot allow emotion to cloud or trump objective judgment.

You need to stand firm, explain your reasoning, and protect the player, no matter what forces of nature are brought to bear—including the wrath of the head coach.

## SUMMARY

Advanced performance is all about the individuality of the athlete, the sport, and the individual position. Taking an athlete from athletic movement to sport and position-specific movements rounds out the plan and ensures the athlete is prepared for the ultimate goal: returning to play.

Sports medicine and sports performance professionals must put egos aside, have the athlete's best interest in mind and come together throughout the process. The athlete must understand the short- and long-term goals and the deadlines for each, so there are no surprises if there is a delay in the return-to-play date.

Having a well thought-out movement analysis and a plan to implement all the required movements will help the athlete achieve the goal of returning to play. This will reduce the chance of re-injury due to unpreparedness for a specific skill required in the sport.

Skills coaches can help ease this transition back to full team participation and improve your knowledge of the sport.

# CHAPTER TWELVE
## BRIDGING THE GAP
## FROM REHAB TO PERFORMANCE—
## FINAL THOUGHTS

There are few things more daunting that returning an athlete to sport. It is a complex process, requiring many moving parts to come together as one whole: the healed athlete performing at the pre-injury state...or better.

That is what motivated me to write this book. I wanted to write a guide where all practitioners, all schools of thought and all training and rehab philosophies are able to meld together into a system that is not dependent on a specific training approach, but on a conceptual continuum where all have their place for the betterment of the athlete.

The aim is for you to apply a patient-focused model that will not only get athletes back to full function, but even more importantly, to full health. We have a moral and ethical obligation to do nothing less.

Often, young professionals ask me about their continuing education path. What should their first course be? What should they focus on next? Seasoned clinicians and strength coaches ask the same question.

By providing the concept of bridging the gap from rehab to performance, I hope

I can answer this question for the individual professional.

If you are someone who, when looking at the continuum, notices you have a lot of education in the fundamental-advancement stage, but minimal experience focusing on somatosensory control, turn back to that section and see some of the areas of study mentioned there so you can seek further continuing education in that area.

You may notice you have a weakness in an area, but your current work situation will not allow you to focus somewhere else. At that point, you know you need to create a professional relationship with someone in field so you can refer your clients out when needed.

We have to stop thinking that our personal area of expertise—whether that is strength and conditioning, athletic training, physical therapy, or any other discipline—is the be-all and end-all when it comes to client care. No matter how good you are and how effective your practice, you simply cannot go it alone.

This book should help you to see where your area of expertise lies, where you need further help, and ultimately where your athletes would benefit when you bring in another expert to focus on a certain area. I hope this book has demonstrated the need for a multidisciplinary team. Anything less is a disservice to our athletes.

As you further your study into certain areas of continuing education, please realize that all schools of thought are saying the same thing. Whether you read the websites of training programs such as FRC, FMS, DNS, or PRI, you will see their fundamental core concepts are similar, for example:

- *Assess your client.*

- *Provide an active intervention.*

- *Reassess your client.*

- *Mobility and stability are important.*

- *The nervous system is important.*

- *The area between the chest and the thighs is important, regardless of the word you use to describe that area.*

- *Breathing will do wonders for the system in everything from survival to relaxation to mobility or stability assistance.*

The core concepts for nearly every worthwhile discipline are similar. They all fit together somewhere along the continuum.

The other thing I hope this book brought to the forefront is the importance of working within a multidisciplinary system. That seems difficult in many situations, but this is a mindset.

You may not be able to employ a nutritionist, but you should have a colleague you can rely on to answer an email or pick up the phone when you call. We should be working with each other *outside* our daily jobs to create interdisciplinary support networks to help us to better bridge the gap from rehab to performance for our athletes.

I hope that as you read this book, you were able to see where your strengths fit in a patient-centered bridging-the-gap model, and that you are also humble enough to see your weaknesses in a new light. This can better inform the gaps in your care strategy and guide you in expanding your network to include professionals who are experts in the skills you do not currently have.

Please look into the references and appendices in the next section for further information on many of these topics. There is simply too much that goes into this continuum to cover one book.

Instead, I hope to have provided a framework in which you can bridge the gap from rehab to performance for your clients, and to have offered even more references for you to refer to for detailed information on other related topics.

One issue with writing a book like this is that information will quickly change. I have tried to provide as many peer-reviewed pieces of literature for your review as I could, however I encourage you to perform your own literature reviews on any topic you find interesting.

The information we have at our fingertips can be overwhelming. Try to stick to systematic reviews and meta-analysis during your lit reviews, and, in the absence of those, randomized controlled trials are helpful.

If you cannot find those, non-randomized controlled trials and case series can provide you with enough information to get you started on a topic.

And, finally, look to scientific principles and your own experience and from those to whom you look up to guide your clinical and strength and conditioning practice.

Bridging the gap from rehab to performance is a complex process. I hope I have begun to do the process justice by presenting an organizational system that will be helpful for decades to come.

It is an exciting time in the realm of sport rehabilitation and sport performance. Information is constantly changing and difficult to keep up with. This organizational system could provide you with a framework for all things old and new, as it relates to progressing an athlete from rehab to performance.

My goal for this book was to provide some structure for you and your colleagues for the betterment of your athletes.

Respectfully and professionally,
Sue Falsone

# APPENDIX LIST

APPENDIX ONE—BRIDGING THE GAP

APPENDIX TWO—THE BRIDGING THE GAP ASSESSMENT

APPENDIX THREE—PAIN, A GUIDE TO CONTRIBUTING MECHANISMS

APPENDIX FOUR—THE JANDA FUNCTIONAL ASSESSMENT

APPENDIX FIVE—THE FMS SCORE SHEET

APPENDIX SIX—THE SFMA SCORE SHEET

APPENDIX SEVEN—TABLE OF ABBREVIATIONS

APPENDIX EIGHT—LIST OF PHOTOS, ILLUSTRATIONS, AND GRAPHICS

APPENDIX NINE—SUGGESTIONS FOR FURTHER STUDY

REFERENCES

INDEX

# APPENDIX ONE
## BRIDGING THE GAP

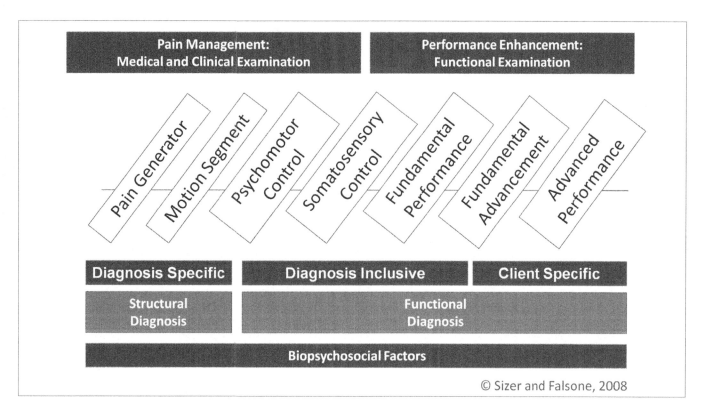

© Sizer and Falsone, 2008

**Pain Generator**
Identifying the tissue that is the issue, if there is one

**Motion Segment**
Identifying the cause of the pain generator

**Psychomotor Control**
Allowing the right muscle to fire at the right time

**Somatosensory Control**
All of the postural reflexes, proprioception, neuromuscular control, and sensorimotor system considerations

**Fundamental Performance**
Foundational strength and power

**Fundamental Advancement**
Athletic movement skill

**Advanced Performance**
Applying athletic movement to a specific sport or task

# APPENDIX TWO
## BRIDGING THE GAP ASSESSMENT

## SAMPLE ONE

| OBJECTIVE DYSFUNCTION | AFFECTS FUNCTION | GOAL | PLAN |
|---|---|---|---|
| 1. FMS Score 8/21 w/ major dysfunctions being in linear and rotational trunk stability, pain in B knees during the deep squat and pain in the L knee during an in-line lunge with his R leg forward. | Poor trunk stability in the linear and rotational directions will significantly affect the way force is transferred from the LE to the UE and can be a major source of his UE and LE issues. Pain at the knees will also limit the ability to transfer force during his pitching motion. | A 12/21 in the functional movement screen in the next four weeks. | Progressive linear and rotational trunk stabilization program, B hip stabilization. |
| 2. Weak iliopsoas, right 3+/5, left 4+/5. Compensatory lumbar motion noted bilaterally. | Weakness and compensatory mvmts for B hip flexion can put add'l stress at other musculatures of the hip. Inability to stabilize the trunk during such movements will also place add'l stress at the hip flexors. This will also affect his ability to transfer force. | 4/5 MMT of B iliopsoas without pain or compensation in four weeks. | Trunk and hip stability; specific iliopsoas strengthening B. |
| 3. Positive scour of the right hip along with anterior pinching at the right hip during end-range hip flexion. R hip IR = 16 degrees. | Possible internal derangement of the R hip along with improper femoral arthrokinematics will give pain and affect the way force is being transferred to the R hip and could increase stress at the R groin. | Negative hip scouring; normalize R hip arthrokinematics in the next four to six weeks. | Joint mobilization to the right hip to normalize hip arthrokinematics. |
| 4. Hip extension mechanics: fatigue of the R glute is noted with over dominant hamstrings. During L hip extension, the B paraspinals kicked in to initiate hip extension motion. | Synergistic dominance will lead to altered mechanics in the way force is transferred from the lower body through the upper body, places add'l stress at the low back and hamstrings. | Normalized muscle firing patterns within four to six weeks. | NMR to bilateral hip and trunk, progressive glute strengthening. |
| 5. Side-lying hip abduction: L initiated movement with his QL, R initiates movements with TFL. | Synergistic dominance will lead to altered to mechanics in the way force is transferred from the lower body through the upper body. | Normalized muscle firing patterns within four to six weeks. | NMR to the R hip with progressive glute strengthening. |

## SAMPLE TWO

| OBJECTIVE DYSFUNCTION | AFFECTS FUNCTION | GOAL | PLAN |
|---|---|---|---|
| 1. Observation: The athlete presents with mild effusion in L knee joint. | 1. Mild effusion my inhibit VMO muscle activity. | 1. Decrease effusion over 4 weeks. | 1. Quad activation and strength, joint mobilization, ice and compression as needed. |
| 2. ROM: L knee flexion 126 degrees, R knee flexion 135 degrees, L knee extension -5 degrees, R knee extension 0 degrees. | 2. Decreased knee ROM will inhibit patient from performing upright load activities. | 2. Normalize pain free ROM in 4-6 weeks. | 2. Joint mobilization to ensure proper joint arthrokinematics for full range of motion. |
| 3. Strength: decreased L lower extremity strength, 4/5, throughout L lower extremity. | 3. Decreased strength will inhibit the muscle's ability to absorb shock and may lead to stress on knee joint. | 3. Normalize pain free strength in 4-6 weeks. | 3. Progressive muscle actvation and strengthening exercises. |

# APPENDIX THREE—PAIN
## A GUIDE TO CONTRIBUTING MECHANISMS

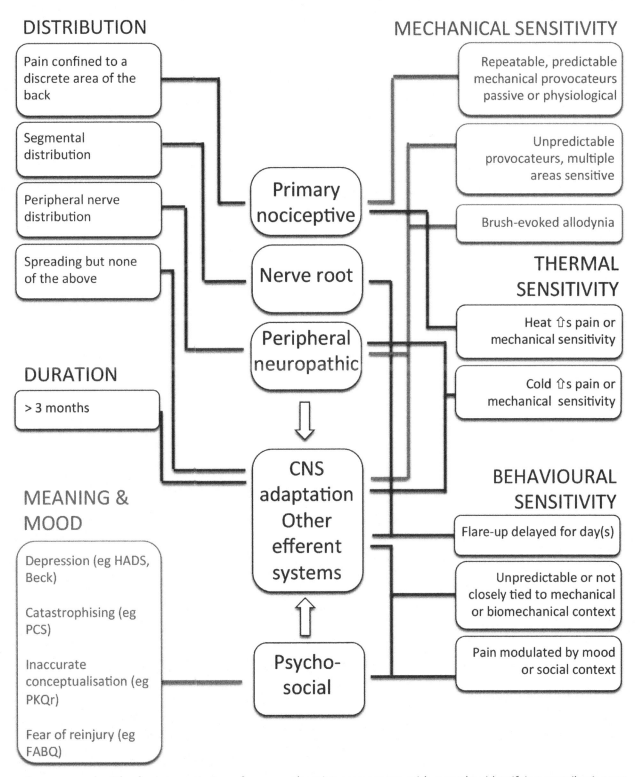

**DISTRIBUTION**

- Pain confined to a discrete area of the back
- Segmental distribution
- Peripheral nerve distribution
- Spreading but none of the above

**MECHANICAL SENSITIVITY**

- Repeatable, predictable mechanical provocateurs passive or physiological
- Unpredictable provocateurs, multiple areas sensitive
- Brush-evoked allodynia

**THERMAL SENSITIVITY**

- Heat ⇧s pain or mechanical sensitivity
- Cold ⇧s pain or mechanical sensitivity

**DURATION**

- > 3 months

**MEANING & MOOD**

- Depression (eg HADS, Beck)
- Catastrophising (eg PCS)
- Inaccurate conceptualisation (eg PKQr)
- Fear of reinjury (eg FABQ)

**BEHAVIOURAL SENSITIVITY**

- Flare-up delayed for day(s)
- Unpredictable or not closely tied to mechanical or biomechanical context
- Pain modulated by mood or social context

Central boxes: Primary nociceptive · Nerve root · Peripheral neuropathic · CNS adaptation Other efferent systems · Psycho-social

Some general guides for interpretation of a comprehensive assessment, with regard to identifying contributions to a pain state from nociceptive and non-nociceptive domains. Patterns are consistent with contribution of biological mechanisms (primary nociceptive, nerve root (also dorsal root ganglion-evoked nociceptive discharge), peripheral neuropathic and central nervous system, immune, autonomic and endocrine contributions). Psychosocial contributions clearly have their effect on the CNS but are not biological contributions. PCS = Pain catastrophising scale; PKQr = Revised pain knowledge questionnaire; FABQ = Fear avoidance beliefs questionnaire.

# APPENDIX FOUR
## JANDA FUNCTIONAL ASSESSMENT
*Copyright JandaApproach.com. Reprinted with permission.*

| | |
|---|---|
| **History and Subjective Complaints** | |
| **Posture—Things to note**<br><br>Muscle tone<br><br>Asymmetry<br><br>Body landmarks | **Observations** |
| **Balance—Things to consider**<br><br>Single-leg stance<br><br>Tandem stance<br><br>Eyes open versus eyes closed<br><br>Head turns | **Observations** |
| **Gait**<br><br>Asymmetry<br><br>Stereotypical patterns | **Observations** |
| **Motor Function—Movement**<br>*(See Assessment and Treatment of Muscle Imbalance, the Janda Approach, Chapter Six for further information)*<br><br>Shoulder abduction<br><br>Push up<br><br>Cervical flexion<br><br>Abdominal curl<br><br>Hib abduction<br><br>Hip extension<br><br>Breath pattern<br><br>Transversus function | **Observations** |

| | |
|---|---|
| **Muscle Length**<br>*(See Assessment and Treatment of Muscle Imbalance, the Janda Approach, Chapter Seven for further information)*<br><br>Upper extremity<br><br>Lower Extremity | **Observations** |
| **Trigger Point Chains**<br>*(See Assessment and Treatment of Muscle Imbalance, the Janda Approach, Chapter Eight for further information)* | **Observations** |
| **Muscle Performance**<br><br>Manual muscle tests as needed | **Testing Results** |
| **Range of Motion—Joint Integrity** | **Results** |
| **Special Tests** | **Record Tests Performed and Results** |
| **Notes** | **Other Objective Findings Not Noted Above** |

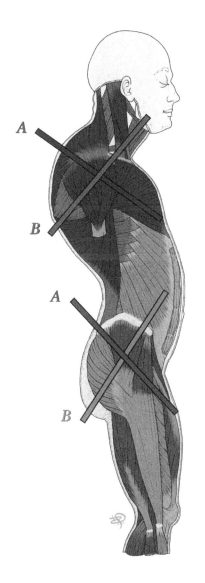

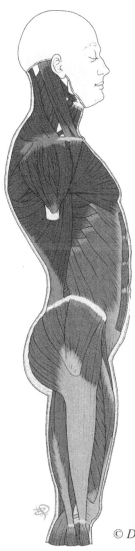

### Muscle Imbalances Associated With
### UPPER CROSSED SYNDROME

| A TIGHT / FACILITATED | B WEAK / INHIBITED |
| --- | --- |
| • Pectoralis | • Longus Capitis |
| • Upper Trapezius | • Longus Colli |
| • Levator Scapula | • Hyoids |
| • Sternocleidomastoid | • Serratus Anterior |
| • Suboccipitals | • Rhomboids |
| • Subscapularis | • Lower Trapezius |
| • Latissimus Dorsi | • Posterior Rotator Cuff |
| • Arm Flexors | • Arm Extensors |

### Muscle Imbalances Associated With
### LOWER CROSSED SYNDROME

| A TIGHT / FACILITATED | B WEAK / INHIBITED |
| --- | --- |
| • Iliopsoas | • Rectus Abdominis |
| • Rectus Femoris | • Transversus Abdominis |
| • Hamstrings | • Obliques |
| • Erector Spinae | • Gluteus Maximus / |
| • Tensor Fascia Lata | • Medius / Minimus |
| • Piriformis | • Vastus Lateralis |
| • Quadratus Lumborum | • Vastus Medialis |
| • Gastroc / Soleus | • Tibialis |

© Danny Quirk

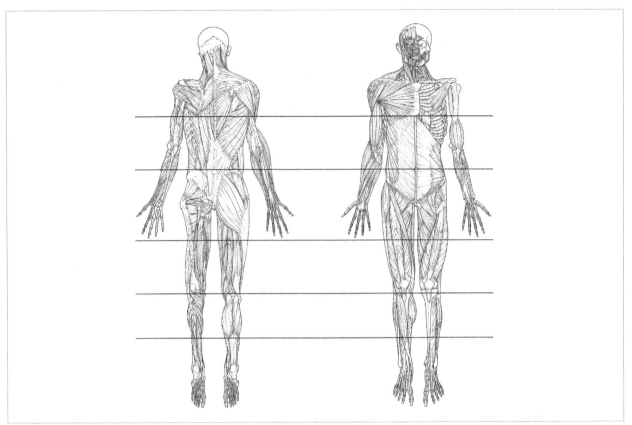

*© Danny Quirk*

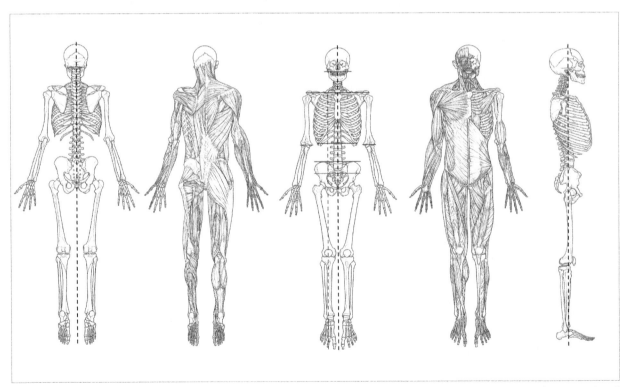

*© Danny Quirk*

# APPENDIX FIVE—FMS SCORE SHEET

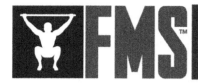 **FUNCTIONAL MOVEMENT SCREEN SCORE SHEET**

NAME: _____ DATE: _____ DOB: _____

ADDRESS: _____

CITY, STATE, ZIP: _____ PHONE: _____

SCHOOL/AFFILIATION: _____

HEIGHT: _____ WEIGHT: _____ AGE: _____ GENDER: _____

PRIMARY SPORT: _____ PRIMARY POSITION: _____

HAND/LEG DOMINANCE: _____ PREVIOUS TEST SCORE: _____

| TEST | | RAW SCORE | FINAL SCORE | COMMENTS |
|---|---|---|---|---|
| DEEP SQUAT | | | | |
| HURDLE STEP | L | | | |
| | R | | | |
| INLINE LUNGE | L | | | |
| | R | | | |
| SHOULDER MOBILITY | L | | | |
| | R | | | |
| SHOULDER CLEARING TEST | L +/- | | | |
| | R +/- | | | |
| ACTIVE STRAIGHT-LEG RAISE | L | | | |
| | R | | | |
| TRUNK STABILITY PUSHUP | | | | |
| EXTENSION CLEARING TEST | +/- | | | |
| ROTARY STABILITY | L | | | |
| | R | | | |
| FLEXION CLEARING TEST | +/- | | | |
| TOTAL SCREEN SCORE | | | | |

Raw Score: This score is used to denote right and left side scoring. The right and left sides are scored in five of the seven tests and both are documented in this space.

Final Score: This score is used to denote the overall score for the test. The lowest score for the raw score (each side) is carried over to give a final score for the test. A person who scores a three on the right and a two on the left would receive a final score of two. The final score is then summarized and used as a total score.

Clearing Test: A positive indicates pain. A negative indicates no pain. If pain is present (+),the score for that test would result in a 0.

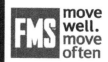 move well. move often

# APPENDIX SIX—THE SFMA SCORE SHEET

## SFMA TOP TIER

| SFMA SCORING | | FN | FP | DP | DN |
|---|---|---|---|---|---|
| Cervical Flexion | | ☐ | ☐ | ☐ | ☐ |
| Cervical Extension | | ☐ | ☐ | ☐ | ☐ |
| Cervical Rotation | L | ☐ | ☐ | ☐ | ☐ |
| | R | ☐ | ☐ | ☐ | ☐ |
| Upper Extremity Pattern 1(MRE) | L | ☐ | ☐ | ☐ | ☐ |
| | R | ☐ | ☐ | ☐ | ☐ |
| Upper Extremity Pattern 2 (LRF) | L | ☐ | ☐ | ☐ | ☐ |
| | R | ☐ | ☐ | ☐ | ☐ |
| Multi-Segmental Flexion | | ☐ | ☐ | ☐ | ☐ |
| Multi-Segmental Extension | | ☐ | ☐ | ☐ | ☐ |
| Multi-Segmental Rotation | L | ☐ | ☐ | ☐ | ☐ |
| | R | ☐ | ☐ | ☐ | ☐ |
| Single-Leg Stance | L | ☐ | ☐ | ☐ | ☐ |
| | R | ☐ | ☐ | ☐ | ☐ |
| Arms Down Deep Squat | | ☐ | ☐ | ☐ | ☐ |

SELECTIVE FUNCTIONAL MOVEMENT ASSESSMENT

SFMA

# SFMA TOP TIER CHECKLIST

**Name:**                    **Date:**              **Total Score:**

**Cervical Flexion**          ☐ Painful
☐ Can't touch sternum to chin
☐ Non-uniform spine curve
☐ Excessive effort and/or lack of motor control

**Cervical Extension**        ☐ Painful
☐ Not within 10 degrees of parallel
☐ Non-uniform spine curve
☐ Excessive effort and/or lack of motor control

**Cervical Rotation**         ☐ Painful Right        ☐ Painful Left
☐ Right      ☐ Left      Chin/Nose not in line with mid-clavicle
☐ Right      ☐ Left      Excessive effort and/or appreciable asymmetry or lack of motor control

**UE Pattern #1 – MRE**       ☐ Painful Right        ☐ Painful Left
☐ Right      ☐ Left      Does not reach inferior angle of scapula
☐ Right      ☐ Left      Excessive effort and/or appreciable asymmetry or lack of motor control

**UE Pattern #2 – LRF**       ☐ Painful Right        ☐ Painful Left
☐ Right      ☐ Left      Does not reach spine of scapula
☐ Right      ☐ Left      Excessive effort and/or appreciable asymmetry or lack of motor control

**Multi-Segmental Flexion**   ☐ Painful
☐ Cannot touch toes
☐ Sacral angle <70 degrees
☐ Non-uniform spine curve
☐ Lack of posterior weight shift
☐ Excessive effort and/or appreciable asymmetry or lack of motor control

**Multi-Segmental Extension**  ☐ Painful
☐ Upper extremity does not achieve or maintain 170
☐ ASIS does not clear toes
☐ Spine of scapula does not clear heels
☐ Non-Uniform spine curve
☐ Excessive effort and/or lack motor control

**Multi-Segmental Rotation**  ☐ Painful Right        ☐ Painful Left
☐ Right      ☐ Left      Pelvis Rotation <50 degrees
☐ Right      ☐ Left      Torso rotation <50 degrees
☐ Right      ☐ Left      Excessive effort and/or lack of symmetry or motor control

**Single-Leg Stance**         ☐ Painful Right        ☐ Painful Left
☐ Right      ☐ Left      Eyes open <10 seconds
☐ Right      ☐ Left      Eyes closed < 10 seconds
☐ Right      ☐ Left      Loss of Height
☐ Right      ☐ Left      Excessive effort or lack of symmetry or motor control

**Arms Down Deep Squat**      ☐ Painful
☐ Hips do not break parallel
☐ Cannot reach fists to ground within footprint
☐ Loss of sagittal plane alignment:    Right_____ Left _____
☐ Excessive effort, weight shift, or motor control

SFMA Certification - Ver 25.6          ©2018 FMS – All rights are reserved.

# APPENDIX SEVEN
## TABLE OF ABBREVIATIONS

| | |
|---|---|
| ACL | Anterior Cruciate Ligament |
| ADL | Activities of daily living |
| AMRAP | As Many Rounds As Possible |
| ART | Active Release Technique |
| AT | Athletic Trainer |
| BOC | Board of Certification |
| CAATE | Commission on Accreditation of Athletic Training Education |
| CNS | Central Nervous System |
| CFSC | Certified Functional Strength Coach |
| COMT | Certified Orthopedic Manual Therapist |
| CRPS | Complex Regional Pain Syndrome |
| CSCS | Certified Strength and Conditioning Specialist |
| DNS | Dynamic Neuromuscular Stabilization |
| DOMS | Delayed Onset Muscle Soreness |
| DPT | Doctor of Physical Therapy |
| DST | Dynamic Systems Theory |
| EXOS | Formally known as Athletes' Performance |
| FAAOMPT | Fellow in the American Academy of Orthopedic Manual Physical Therapy |
| FMS | Functional Movement Screen |
| FRC | Functional Range Conditioning |
| GERD | Gastroesophageal Reflux Disease |
| HA | Hyaluronan or Hyluronic Acid |
| IASTM | Instrument-Assisted Soft Tissue Mobilization |
| ISS | Integrated Stabilizing System |
| IYCA | International Youth Conditioning Association |
| KT | Kinesiology Tape |
| MAT | Muscle Activation Technique |

| | |
|---|---|
| MD | Medical doctor |
| MSI | Movement System Impairment |
| NCM | Non-Counter Movements |
| NSLBP | Non-Specific Low Back Pain |
| PAG | Periaqueductal gray matter |
| PNF | Proprioceptive Neuromuscular Facilitation |
| PNS | Peripheral Nervous System |
| PRI | Postural Restoration Institute |
| PT | Physical Therapist |
| RICE | Rest, Ice, Compression, Elevation |
| SFMA | Selective Functional Movement Assessment |
| SCCC | Strength and Conditioning Coach Certified |
| SMS | Sensorimotor system |
| TCM | Traditional Chinese Medicine |
| TENS | Transcutaneous Electrical Nerve Stimulation |
| TL | Thoracolumbar (junction) |
| TRX | Suspension training equipment |
| VAS | Visual Analog Scale |

# APPENDIX EIGHT
## LIST OF PHOTOS,
## ILLUSTRATIONS, AND GRAPHICS

### ILLUSTRATIONS AND GRAPHICS

## PHOTOGRAPHS

# APPENDIX NINE
## SUGGESTIONS FOR FURTHER STUDY

**acatoday.org**

The website for the largest professional chiropractic association in the US

**acsm.org**

The American College of Sports Medicine is the largest sports medicine and exercise science organization in the world

**ama-assn.org**

The official website of the American Medical Association

**americanweightlifting.com**

Olympic weightlifting coach Glenn Pendlay's site

**anatomytrains.com/kmi**

The Anatomy Trains website, highlighting the work of Tom Myers

**apta.org**

The American Physical Therapy Association is an individual membership professional organization for physical therapists

**apta.org/StateIssues/DirectAccess**

For further information on direct access to physical therapy in your state

**atsu.edu**

A.T. Still University is the founding institution for osteopathic healthcare, founded in 1892 by Andrew Taylor Still

**bmulligan.com**

The website for Brian Mulligan and his mobilization with movement manual therapy techniques

**bocatc.org**

The board of certification is the credentialing agency who provides a certification program for the entry level athletic training professional

**bodybyboyle.com**

Michael Boyle's strength and conditioning facility website

**brandonmarcellophd.com**

Brandon Marcello's official website for high performance

**buckeyeperformancegolf.com**

For information related to fitness, performance, assessment, and rehabilitation

**certifiedfsc.com**

The website for the Certified Functional Strength Coach, the strength and conditioning certification by Michael Boyle

**coachdos.com**

Robert dos Remedios' website for strength and conditioning

**cvilleneuroandsleep.com**

Chris Winter's website for the Charlottesville Neurology and Sleep Medicine clinic

**danjohn.net**

The official website for Dan John—athlete, strength coach, and author

**facebook.com/dannyquirkartwork**

Danny Quirk, medical illustrator for *Bridging the Gap from Rehab to Performance*

**fascial-fitness.de/en/starting-page**

The website for fascial fitness, the original training method for fascial training

**fascialmanipulation.com/en/**

The website for Fascial Manipulation, created by Luigi Stecco

**functionalanatomyseminars.com**

For further information on Functional Range Release, Functional Range Conditioning, and Functional Range Assessment

**functionalmovement.com**

The website for the Functional Movement System, including the FMS, SFMA, YBT, and FCS

**functionalmovement.com/system/sfma**

For information related to the Selective Functional Movement Assessment

**goldmedalmind.net**

Dr. Jim Afremow's website, featuring his book *The Champion's Comeback*

**graycook.com**

Gray Cook's article and podcast website

**hawkgrips.com**

HawkGrips official website for Instrument Assisted Soft Tissue Mobilization

**hevatech.com**

For further information on cupping therapy and cupping instruments

**immaculatedissection**

Anatomy teaching site by Danny Quirk, Kathy Dooley, and Anna Folckomer

**iyca.org**

The website for the International Youth Conditioning Association

**jandaapproach.com**

For further information on the work of Dr. Vladimir Janda

**meyerpt.com**

For health care related products and equipment

**mobilitywod.com**

Kelly Starrett's website, the Mobility WOD

*mohrresults.com*

Chris and Kara Mohr's website for nutritional and lifestyle information

*muscleactivation.com*

The official website for Muscle Activation Techniques® for muscle imbalances

*mytpi.com*

For golf-specific health, fitness, and swing advice

*nata.org*

The National Athletic Trainers' Association is the professional membership association for certified athletic trainers

*nata.org/about/athletic-training/obtain-certification*

For further information on how to become a Certified Athletic Trainer

*nsca.com*

The National Strength and Conditioning Association is a membership organization for strength coaches, personal trainers, researchers, and educators in the strength and conditioning field

*nsca.com/Certification/CSCS*

For further information on thhe NSCA certification called the Certified Strength and Conditioning Specialist

*olagrimsby.com*

The website for the Ola Grimsby Institute

*onebyonenutrition.com*

For further information on nutrition and weight loss

*otpbooks.com*

For books, videos and audio lectures related to strength and conditioning and physical medicine

*performbetter.com*

For equipment needs, facility design, and continuing education

*phillipbeach.com*

Phillip Beach's website, author of *Muscles and Meridians*

*pilates.com/BBAPP/V/index.html*

Balance Body's website for further information on Pilates and Pilates-related products and education

*posturalrestoration.com*

The official website for the Postural Restoration Institute

*powerplate.com*

For further information on vibrational training and products

*powerspeedendurance.com*

Power Speed Endurance is a programming, coaching, and educational platform for developing sports performance, fitness, and health

**precisionnutrition.com**

For further information on nutrition

**pt.wustl.edu/education/movement-system-impairment-syndromes-courses**

Information on Movement System Impairments developed by Shirley Sahrmann

**rehabps.com/REHABILITATION/Home.html**

For further information on the Prague School and Dynamic Neuromuscular Stabilization

**rolf.org/history.php**

For further information on Ida Rolf, the Rolf Institute and Rolfing Structural Integration

**somatics.de/en**

The official website for Robert Schleip, known for his work in the field of fascia

**squattypotty.com**

The toilet stool

**strengthcoach.com**

Michael Boyle's strength coach forum and education website

**strongfirst.com**

For information on Pavel Tsatsouline, kettlebell, and strength training education

**structureandfunction.net**

My education company and for further information on dry needling and cupping

**suefalsone.com**

My website

**teamexos.com**

The official website for EXOS

**thesleepsolutionbook.com**

For more information on Dr. Chris Winter's sleep book

**trxtraining.com**

For further information on suspension training and products

**tuneupfitness.com**

Jill Miller's website and information on the Roll Model® and Yoga Tune Up®

**upledger.com/therapies/faq.php**

For further information on Craniosacral Therapy

**wilfleming.com**

Wil Fleming's website for Olympic lifting education and coaching

**yogaalliance.org**

For further information on yoga teacher training

**yogatoes.com**

The website for the product Yoga Toes

# APPENDIX TEN
## REFERENCES

*Note: Ibid means "same as previous."*

[1] Athletic Trainers, Regulation and Credentials, *www.nata.org/about/athletic-training*

[2] William Kuchera and Michael Kuchera, *Osteopathic Principles in Practice.*

[3] Andrew J. Teichtahl et al, "Wolff's Law in Action: a Mechanism for Early Knee Otearthritis," Arthritis Research and Therapy, September 2015.

[4] Paul W. Hodges, Kylie Tucker, "Moving Differently in Pain: A New Theory to Explain the Adaptation to Pain," *Pain,* 2011.

[5] Leeuw M, Goossens MEJB, Linton SJ, Crombez G, Boersma K, Vlaeyen JWS, "The Fear-Avoidance Model of Musculo-skeletal Pain: Current State of Scientific Evidence," *Journal of Behavioral Medicine,* 2007;30(1):77-94.doi:10.1007/s10865-006-9085-0.

[6] Hug F, Hodges PW, Tucker K, "Task dependency of motor adaptations to an acute noxious stimulation," *Journal of Neurophysiology,* 2014;111(11):2298-2306.doi:10.1152/jn.00911.2013.

[7] Hug F, Hodges PW, Carroll TJ, De Martino E, Magnard J, Tucker K, "Motor Adaptations to Pain during a Bilateral Plantarflexion Task: Does the Cost of Using the Non-Painful Limb Matter?" *PLOS ONE,* 2016;11(4):e0154524.

[8] Hug F, Hodges PW, Carroll TJ, De Martino E, Magnard J, Tucker K, (2016) Motor Adaptations to Pain during Biateral Plantarflexion Task: Does the Cost of Using the Non-Painful Limb Matter? *PLOS ONE,* 11(4):e0154524.doi:10.1371/journal.pone.0154524.

[9] Covassin T, Beidler E, Ostrowski J, Wallace J, "Psychosocial Aspects of Rehabilitation in Sports," *Clinics in Sports Medicine,* 2015;34(2):199-212.doi:10.1016/j.csm.2014.12.004.

[10] Page P, Frank C, Lardner R, *Assessment And Treatment Of Muscle Imbalance, 1st edition,* Champaign, IL, Human Kinetics, 2010.

[11] Mark D. Thelen et al, "The Clinical Efficacy of Kinesio Tape for Shoulder Pain," *Journal of Orthopedic and Sports Physical Therapy,* 2008.

[12] Hug F, Hodges PW, Carroll TJ, De Martino E, Magnard J, Tucker K, "Motor Adaptations to Pain during a Bilateral Plantarflexion Task: Does the Cost of Using the Non-Painful Limb Matter?" *PLOS ONE,* 2016;11(4):e0154524.

[13] TL Chmielewski, "The Association of Pain and Fear of Movement/Re-injury with Function During Anterior Cruciate Ligament Reconstruction Rehabilitation," *Journal of Orthopedic Sports Physical Therapy,* December 2008.

[14] Leeuw M, Goossens MEJB, Linton SJ, Crombez G, Boersma K, Vlaeyen JWS, "The Fear-Avoidance Model of Musculo-skeletal Pain: Current State of Scientific Evidence," *Journal of Behavioral Medicine,* 2007;30(1):77-94.doi:10.1007/s10865-006-9085-0.

[15] Stecco L, *Fascial Manipulation For Muscuskeletal Pain, 1st edition,* Padova, Italy, Piccin Nuova Libraria S. P. A, 2004.

[16] Swanson RL, "Biotensegrity: a unifying theory of biological architecture with applications to osteopathic practice, education, and research—a review and analysis," *Journal of the American Osteopathic Association,* 2013;113(1):34–52.

[17] Paul W. Hodges and Carolyn A. Richardson, "Insufficient Muscular Stabilization of the Lumbar Spine Associated with Low Back Pain," *SPINE,* 1996.

[18] Papadimitriou G, "The 'Biopsychosocial Model': 40 years of application in Psychiatry," *Psychiatrki,* 2017;28(2):107-110.doi:10.22365/jpsych.2017.282.107.

[19] Dario Riva et al, "Proprioceptive Training and Injury Prevention in a Professional Men's Basketball Team: A Six-Year Prospective Study," *Journal of Strength and Conditioning Research,* February 2016.

[20] Ibid.

[21] Gray Cook, "The Art of Screening, Part 2: Failure, Feedback and Success," *graycook.com.*

[22] K. E. Wilk et al, "Rehabilitation of the Overhead Athlete's Elbow," *Sports Health,* September 2012.

[23] Kendall F, McCreary, E. *Muscles, 5th edition,* Baltimore, MD, Lippincott Williams & Wilkins, 2005.

[24] Robert C. Manske, *Postsurgical Orthopedic Sports Rehabilitation: Knee and Shoulder,* 171-173.

[25] Thomas Haugen et al, "Effects of Core-Stability Training on Performance and Injuries in Competitive Athletes," *Sport Science,* 2016.

[26] Gregory D, Myer et al, "Rehabilitation After Anterior Cruciate Ligament Reconstruction: Criteria-Based Progression Through the Return-to-Sport Phase," *Journal of Orthopedic and Sports Physical Therapy,* 2006.

[27] Sheri Walters, "When to Progress, When to Regress," *Perform Better,* available online at http://www.performbetter.com/webapp/wcs/stores/servlet/PBOnePieceView?storeId=10151andcatalogId=10751andpagename=550.

[28] R Nahin, "Estimates of Pain Prevalence and Severity in Adults: United States 2012," *The Journal of Pain,* Vol 16, No 8 (August), 2015.

[29] Ibid.

[30] M. Moayedi and K. D. Davis, "Theories of Pain: From Specificity to Gate Control," *Journal of Neurophysiology,* 2013;109(1):5-12. doi:10.1152/jn.00457.2012.

[31] Ibid.

[32] Cagnie B, Dewitte V, Barbe T, Timmermans F, Delrue N, Meeus M, "Physiologic Effects of Dry Needling," *Current Pain Headache Reports,* 2013;17(8). doi:10.1007/s11916-013-0348-5.

[33] R. Melzack, "Pain and the Neuromatrix in the Brain," *Journal of Dental Education,* 2001.

[34] Moseley, Lorimer, *Pain,* 978-193104657, On Target Publications, March 2015.

[35] International Association for the Study of Pain definition of Pain

http://www.iasp-pain.org/Taxonomy?navItemNumber=576#Pain, Accessed 2/19/2018

[36] G. DelForge, *Musculoskeletal Trauma: Implications for Sports Injury Management.*

[37] Adam Gopnik, "Feel Me: What The Science of Touch Says About Ourselves," *The New Yorker,* May 2016.

[38] Hug F, Hodges PW, Carroll TJ, De Martino E, Magnard J, Tucker K, "Motor Adaptations to Pain during a Bilateral Plantarflexion Task: Does the Cost of Using the Non-Painful Limb Matter?" *PLOS ONE,* 2016;11(4):e0154524.

[39] Francois Hug et al, "Motor Adaptations to Pain during a Bilateral Plantarflexion Task: Does the Cost of Using the Non-Painful Limb Matter?" *PLOS ONE,* April 2016.

[40] Qaseem A, Wilt TJ, McLean RM, Forciea MA, for the Clinical Guidelines Committee of the American College of Physicians, "Noninvasive Treatments for Acute, Subacute, and Chronic Low Back Pain: A Clinical Practice Guideline From the American College of Physicians," *Annals of Internal Medicine,* 2017;166(7):514.doi:10.7326/M16-2367.

[41] Gabe Mirkin, "Why Ice Delays Recovery," April 2013, available online at http://www.drmirkin. com/fitness/why-ice-delays-recovery. html.

[42] Van den Bekerom MP, Struijs PA, Blankevoort L, Welling L, Van Dijk CN, Kerkhoffs GM, "What is the evidence for rest, ice, compression, and elevation therapy in the treatment of ankle sprains in adults?" *Journal of Athletic Training,* 2012;47(4):435–443.

[43] F. R. Noyes, "Functional Properties of Knee Ligaments and Alterations Induced by Immobilization: A Correlative Biomechanical and Histological Study in Primates," *Clinical Orthopedics and Related Research,* 1977; S. L. Woo et al, "The Biomechanical and Morphological Changes in the Medial Collateral Ligament of the Rabbit after Immobilization and Remobilization," *The Journal of Bone and Joint Surgery,* 1987.

[44] TAH Jarvinen, "Muscle Injuries: Biology and Treatment," *American Journal of Sports Medicine,* 2005.

[45] Bahram Jam, "Paradigm Shifts: Use of Ice and NSAIDs Post-Acute Soft Tissue Injuries," Advanced Physical Therapy Institute.

[46] Nicolas J Pillon et al, "Cross-talk Between Skeletal Muscle and Immune Cells: Muscle-Derived Mediators and Metabolic Implications," *American Journal of Physiology—Endocrinology and Metabolism,* March 2013.

[47] Melzack R, Wall P, "Pain Mechanisms: A New Theory," 1965;150(3699):971-979.

[48] M. A. Merrick, "Secondary Injury After Musculoskeletal Trauma: A Review and Update," *Journal of Athletic Training,* 2002; M. A. Merrick MA and N. M. McBrier, "Progression of Secondary Injury after Musculoskeletal Trauma: A Window of Opportunity?" *Journal of Sports Rehabilitation,* 2010.

[49] Bleakley CM, Glasgow P, Webb MJ, "Cooling an acute muscle injury: can basic scientific theory translate into the clinical setting?" *British Journal of Sports Medicine,* 2012;46(4):296-298.

[50] Merrick MA, "Secondary injury after musculoskeletal trauma: a review and update." *Journal of Athletic Training,* 2002;37(2):209.

[51] Merrick MA, Rankin JM, Andres FA, et al, "A preliminary examination of cryotherapy and secondary injury in skeletal muscle," *Medicine & Science in Sports & Exercise, 1999;31:1516–21.*

[52] Myrer WJ, Myrer KA, Measom GJ, et al, "Muscle Temperature Is Affected by Overlying Adipose When Cryotherapy Is Administered," *Journal of Athletic Training, 2001;36:32–6.*

[53] TJ Hubbard and Craig R. Denegar, "Does Cryotherapy Improve Outcomes with Soft Tissue Injury," *American Journal of Sports Medicine,* 2004.

[54] KKW Tsang et al, "Volume Decreases After Elevation and Intermittent Compression of Post-acute Ankle Sprains Are Negated by Gravity-Dependent Positioning," *Journal of Athletic Training,* 2003.

[55] Zhou, K, Ma, Y, and Brogan, MS, "Dry needling versus acupuncture: the ongoing debate," *Acupuncture in Medicine Journal of the British Medical Acupuncture Society,* 2015.

[56] Karl Lewit, "The Needle Effect in the Relief of Myofascial Pain," *Pain,* 1979.

[57] R. Butts et al, "Peripheral and Spinal Mechanisms of Pain and Dry Needling Mediated Analgesia: A Clinical Resource Guide for Health Care Professionals," *International Journal of Physical Medicine Rehabilitation*, 2016; B. Cagnie et al, "Physiologic Effects of Dry Needling," *Current Pain and Headache Reports*, 2013.

[58] B. Cagnie et al, "Physiologic Effects of Dry Needling," *Current Pain and Headache Reports*, 2013.

[59] Melzack R, Wall P, "Pain Mechanisms: A New Theory," 1965;150(3699):971-979.

[60] Cagnie B, Dewitte V, Barbe T, Timmermans F, Delrue N, Meeus M, "Physiologic Effects of Dry Needling," *Current Pain and Headache Reports,* 2013;17(8).doi:10.1007/s11916-013-0348-5.

[61] Moayedi M, Davis KD, "Theories of pain: from specificity to gate control," *Journal of Neurophysiology,* 2013;109(1):5-12.doi:10.1152/jn.00457.2012.

[62] Ibid.

[63] DM Kietrys, "Effectiveness of Dry Needling for Upper-Quarter Myofascial Pain: A Systematic Review and Meta-Analysis," *Journal of Orthopedic Sports Physical Therapy,* Sept 2013.

[64] Jan Dommerholt, "Dry Needling—Peripheral and Central Considerations," *The Journal of Manual and Manipulative Therapy*, Nov 2011.

[65] Bandy W, Nelson R, Beamer L, "Comparison of Dry Needling vs. Sham on The Performance of Vertical Jump," *International Journal of Sports Physical Therapy,* 2017;12(5):747-751.

[66] Haser C, StöGgl T, Kriner M, et al, "Effect of Dry Needling on Thigh Muscle Strength and Hip Flexion in Elite Soccer Players," *Medicine & Science in Sports & Exercise*, 2017;49(2):378-383.doi:10.1249/MSS.0000000000001111.

[67] Caramagno J, Adrian L, Mueller L, Purl J, "Analysis of Competencies for Dry Needling by Physical Therapists," https://www.fsbpt.org/Portals/0/documents/free-resources/DryNeedlingFinalReport_20150812.pdf, accessed July 30, 2016.

[68] B. Cagnie et al, "Physiologic Effects of Dry Needling," *Current Pain and Headache Reports*, 2013; R. Butts et al, "Peripheral and Spinal Mechanisms of Pain and Dry Needling Mediated Analgesia: A Clinical Resource Guide for Health Care Professionals," *International Journal of Physical Medicine Rehabilitation*, 2016; L. W. Chou et al, "Probable Mechanisms of Needling Therapies for Myofascial Pain Control," *Evidence-Based Complementary Alternative Medicine*, 2012; J. Dunning et al, "Dry needling: a Literature Review with Implications for Clinical Practice Guidelines," *Physical Therapy Review*, 2014.

[69] Barbara Cagnie et al, "Physiologic Effects of Dry Needling," *Current Pain and Headache Reports,* 2013.

[70] Melzack R, Wall P, "Pain Mechanisms: A New Theory," 1965;150(3699):971-979.

[71] Bilgili A, Çakır T, Doğan ŞK, Erçalık T, Filiz MB, Toraman F, "The effectiveness of transcutaneous electrical nerve stimulation in the management of patients with complex regional pain syndrome: A randomized, double-blinded, placebo-controlled prospective study," *Journal of Back Musculoskeletal Rehabilitation*, 2016;29(4):661-671.doi:10.3233/BMR-160667.

[72] Draper D, Prentice W, "Chapter 4. Therapeutic Ultrasound," *Therapeutic Modalities in Rehabilitation, Fourth Edition*, Access Physiotherapy, McGraw-Hill Medical, http://accessphysiotherapy.mhmedical.com.p.atsu.edu/content/aspx?bookid=465&sectionid=40195349. Accessed June 8, 2017.

[73] Kalron 2003, Lim 2015, Montalvo 2014, Morris 2013, Taylor 2014, Williams 2012.

[74] DH Craighead et al, "Kinesiology Tape Increases Cutaneous Microvascular Blood Flow Independent of Tape Tension," *17th Annual TRAC Conference*, 2015.

[75] Edwin Lim and Matthew Tay, "Kinesio Taping in Musculoskeletal Pain and Disability that Lasts for More Than 4 Weeks: It is Time to Peel Off the Tape and Throw It Out With The Sweat?" *British Journal of Sports Medicine*, 2015.

[76] Craighead et al, "Topical Menthol Application Augments Cutaneous Microvascular Blood Flow," *International Journal of Exercise Science*, 2016.

[77] Pramod Johar et al, "A Comparison of Topical Menthol to Ice on Pain, Evoked Tetanic and Voluntary Force During Delayed Onset Muscle Soreness," *Journal of Sports Physical Therapy,* 2012.

[78] Susanna Stea et al, "Essential Oils for Complementary Treatment of Surgical Patients: State of the Art," *Evidence-Based Complementary and Alternative Medicine*, 2014.

[79] Yang Suk Yun et al, "Effect of Eucalyptus Oil Inhalation on Pain and Inflammatory Responses after Total Knee Replacement: A Randomized Clinical Trial," *Evidence-Based Complementary and Alternative Medicine*, 2013.

[80] Hug F, Hodges PW, Carroll TJ, De Martino E, Magnard J, Tucker K, "Motor Adaptations to Pain during a Bilateral Plantarflexion Task: Does the Cost of Using the Non-Painful Limb Matter?" *PLOS ONE,* 2016;11(4):e0154524.

[81] Beardsley C, Contreras B, "The functional movement screen: A review," *Strength & Conditioning Journal*, 2014;36(5):72–80.

[82] Ibid.

[83] Frost DM, Beach TA, Callaghan JP, McGill SM, "FMS Scores Change With Performers' Knowledge of the Grading Criteria—Are General Whole-Body Movement Screens Capturing 'Dysfunction'?" *Journal of Strength & Conditioning Research,* 2015;29(11):3037–3044.

[84] Glaws K, Juneau C, Becker L, Di Stasi S, Hewett TE, "Intra- and Inter- Rater Reliability of the Selective Functional Movement Assessment (SFMA)," *International Journal of Sports Physical Therapy*, 2014;9(2):195-207.

85 Page P, Frank C, Lardner R, *Assessment and Treatment of Muscle Imbalance: The Janda Approach*, Human Kinetics, Champaign, IL, 2010.

86 Hoogenboom BJ, Voight ML, "Clinical commentary rolling revisited: using rolling to assess and treat neuromuscular control and coordination of the core and extremities of athletes," *International Journal of Sports Physical Therapy*, 2015;10(6):787-802.

87 Rosário JL, "Biomechanical assessment of human posture: a literature review," *Journal of Bodywork Movement Therapies*, 2014;18(3):368-373.doi:10.1016/j.jbmt.2013.11.018.

88 Page P, Frank C, Lardner R, *Assessment and Treatment of Muscle Imbalance: The Janda Approach*, Human Kinetics, Champaign, IL, 2010.

89 Kendall, Florence Peterson, *Muscles: Testing And Function With Posture And Pain*, Baltimore, MD, Lippincott Williams & Wilkins, 2005.

90 Brian Mulligan, www.brian-mulligan.com.

91 Stanley Paris, www.spine-health.com/doctor/physical-therapist/stanley-paris-st-augustine-fl.

92 Ola Grimsby, www.olagrimsby.com.

93 Carla Stecco, *Functional Atlas of the Human Fascial System*, 2015

94 Ibid.

95 Ibid.

96 Ibid.

97 Findley T, Chaudhry H, Dhar S, "Transmission of muscle force to fascia during exercise," *Journal of Bodywork Movement Therapies*, 2015;19(1):119-123. doi:10.1016/j.jbmt.2014.08.010.

98 Seunghun Lee, MD, Kyung Bin Joo, MD, Soon-Young Song, MD, "Accurate Definition of Superficial and Deep Fascia," *Radiology*, December 2011.

99 Michael Seffinger, "Abdominal Visceral Manipulation Prevents and Reduces Peritoneal Adhesions," *Journal of the American Osteopathic Association*, January 2013.

100 Findley T, Chaudhry H, Dhar S, "Transmission of muscle force to fascia during exercise," *Journal of Bodywork Movement Therapies*, 2015;19(1):119-123.doi:10.1016/j.jbmt.2014.08.010.

101 Fascial manipulation, www.fascialmanipulation.com/en/about-fascial-manipulation. aspx?lang=en

102 Stecco L, *Fascial Manipulation for Musculoskeletal Pain*, Piccin-Nuova Libraria, 2012.

103 Mike Reinold, "Fascial Manipulation," www.mikereinold.com/

104 Stecco C, Stern R, Porzionato A, et al, "Hyaluronan within fascia in the etiology of myofascial pain," *Surgical and Radiologic Anatomy*, 2011;33(10):891-896.doi:10.1007/s00276-011-0876-9.

105 Stecco C, Stern R, Porzionato A, et al, "Hyaluronan within fascia in the etiology of myofascial pain," *Surgical and Radiologic Anatomy*, 2011;33(10):891-896.doi:10.1007/s00276-011-0876-9.

106 C. Stecco et al, "Hyaluronan within fascia in the etiology of myofascial pain," *Surgical and Radiologic Anatomy*, 2011.

107 Delforge, G, *Musculskeletal Trauma: Implications for Sports Injury Management*, Champaign, IL, Human Kinetics, 2002.

108 C. Stecco et al, "Hyaluronan within fascia in the etiology of myofascial pain," *Surgical and Radiologic Anatomy*, 2011.

109 Matteini P, Dei L, Carretti E, Volpi N, Goti A, Pini R, "Structural Behavior of Highly Concentrated Hyaluronan," *Biomacromolecules*, 2009;10(6):1516-1522. doi:10.1021/bm900108z.

110 Carla and Antonio Stecco et al, "Analysis of the Presence of the Hyaluronic Acid Inside the Deep Fasciae and in the Muscles," *Italian Journal of Anatomy and Embryology*, North America, November 2011.

111 Thomas Myers, "A Brief History of Anatomy Trains," www.anatomytrains.com/about-us/history/

112 Krause F, Wilke J, Vogt L, Banzer W, "Intermuscular force transmission along myofascial chains: a systematic review," *Journal of Anatomy*, 2016;228(6):910-918.doi:10.1111/joa.12464.

113 Robert Schleip, "Fascial Plasticity—A New Neurobiological Explanation, Part II," *Journal of Bodywork and Movement Therapies*, April 2003.

114 Tozzi P, "A unifying neuro-fasciagenic model of somatic dysfunction—Underlying mechanisms and treatment, Part II," *Journal of Bodywork and Movement Therapies*, 2015;19(3):526-543.doi:10.1016/j.jbmt.2015.03.002.

115 Stecco C, Porzionato A, Macchi V et al, "A histological study of the deep fascia of the upper limb," *Italian Journal of Anatomy and Embryology*, 2006;111:105–10.

116 Robert Schleip, *Fascia in Sport and Movement*.

117 Thomas Myers, "Fascial Fitness Resources," www.fascialfitnesstoday.com.

118 Vagus nerve anatomy: http://emedicine.medscape.com/article/1875813-overview

119 Jill Miller, *The Roll Model*, 159-161.

120 Mark Butler, "Deep Impact," provided courtesy of HawkGrips.

[121] Warren Hammer, "New Research Regarding Instrument-Assisted Soft-Tissue Mobilization," *Dynamic Chiropractic,* May 2008.

[122] Khan KM, "Mechanotherapy: how physical therapists' prescription of exercise promotes tissue repair," *British Journal of Sports Medicine,* 2009;43(4):247-252.

[123] MT Loghmani et al, "Instrument-Assisted Cross-Fiber Massage Accelerates Knee Ligament Healing," *Journal of Orthopedic Sports Physical Therapy,* 2006.

[124] Janet McMurray et al, "A Comparison and Review of Indirect Myofascial Release Therapy, Instrument-Assisted Soft Tissue Mobilization, and Active Release Techniques to Inform Clinical Decision Making," *International Journal of Athletic Therapy and Training,* November 2015.

[125] Andrea Portillo-Soto et al, "Comparison of Blood Flow Changes with Soft Tissue Mobilization and Massage Therapy," *The Journal of Alternative and Complementary Medicine,* 2014.

[126] Robert Schleip et al, "Strain Hardening of Fascia: Static Stretching of Dense Fibrous Connective Tissues can Induce a Temporary Stiffness Increase Accompanied by Enhanced Matrix Hydration," *Journal of Bodywork and Movement Therapies, 2011.*

[127] Anthony Carey, "Myofascial Mobility Through Strategic Movement," *PT on the Net,* June 2012.

[128] Veli-PekkaSipila, "The Rationale for Joint Mobilization as a Manual Technique," http://www. orthosportonline. com/.

[129] Huber R, Emerich M, Braeunig M, "Cupping— Is it reproducible? Experiments about factors determining the vacuum," *Complementary Therapies in Medicine,* 2011;19(2):78-83.

[130] El Sayed et al, "Medical and Scientific Bases of Wet Cupping Therapy (Al-hijamah): in Light of Modern Medicine and Prophetic Medicine," *Alternative Integrated Medicine,* 2013.

[131] Lauche R, Cramer H, Hohmann C, et al. The Effect of Traditional Cupping on Pain and Mechanical Thresholds in Patients with Chronic Nonspecific Neck Pain: A Randomised Controlled Pilot Study, *Evidence Based Complementary Alternative Medicine,* 2012;2012:1-10.doi:10.1155/2012/429718.

[132] Rozenfeld E, Kalichman L, "New is the well-forgotten old: The use of dry cupping in musculoskeletal medicine," *Journal of Bodywork and Movement Therapies,* 2016;20(1):173-178.

[133] Huber R, Emerich M, Braeunig M, "Cupping—It is reproducible? Experiments about factors determining the vacuum," *Complementary Therapies in Medicine,* 2011;19(2):78-83.doi:10.1016/j.ctim.2010.12.006.

[134] Tham LM, Lee HP, Lu C, "Cupping: From a biomechanical perspective," *Journal of Biomechanics,* 2006;39(12):2183-2193.doi:10.1016/j.jbiomech.2005.06.027.

[135] Kim J-I, Lee MS, Lee D-H, Boddy K, Ernst E, "Cupping for Treating Pain: A Systematic Review," *Evidence Based Complementary Alternative Medicine,* 2011;2011:1-7.doi:10.1093/ecam/nep035.

[136] Cao H, Han M, Li X et al, "Clinical research evidence of cupping therapy in China: a systematic literature review," *BMC Complementary and Alternative Medicine,* 2010;10(1):70.

[137] Tham LM, Lee HP, Lu C, "Cupping: From a biomechanical perspective," *Journal of Biomechanics,* 2006;39(12):2183-2193

[138] Istrătoaie O, Pirici I, Ofiţeru A-M et al, "Evaluation of cardiac microvasculature in patients with diffuse myocardial fibrosis," *Romanian Journal of Morphology and Embryology,* 2016;57(4):1351.

[139] Coderre TJ, Bennett GJ, "A hypothesis for the cause of complex regional pain syndrome-type I (reflex sympathetic dystrophy): pain due to deep-tissue microvascular pathology," *Pain Medicine Malden Mass,* 2010;11(8):1224-1238.

[140] Ibid.

[141] Gary Delforge, *Musculoskeletal Trauma: Implications for Sports Injury Management.*

[142] E. H. Shin et al, "Quality of Healing: Defining, Quantifying, and Enhancing Skeletal Muscle Healing: Muscle Injury Repair and Regeneration," *Wound Repair Regeneration,* 2014.

[143] MS Lee, "Cupping for Hypertension: A Systematic Review," *Clinical and Experimental Hypertension,* 2010.

[144] Walker SC, Trotter PD, Swaney WT, Marshall A, Mcglone FP, "C-tactile afferents: Cutaneous mediators of oxytocin release during affiliative tactile interactions?" *Neuropeptides,* January 2017.

[145] Marzieh Akbarzade, "Comparison of the Effect of Dry Cupping Therapy and Acupressure at BL23 Point on Intensity of Postpartum Perineal Pain Based on the Short Form of McGill Pain Questionnaire," *Journal of Reproductive and Infertility,* Jan-March 2016.

[146] Huijuan Caoa et al, "An Overview of Systematic Reviews of Clinical Evidence for Cupping Therapy," *Journal of Traditional Chinese Medical Sciences,* 2015.

[147] Robert Schleip, *Fascia in Sport and Movement*; Thomas W. Myers, *Anatomy Trains: Myofascial Meridians for Manual and Movement Therapists;* Carla Stecco, *Functional Atlas of the Human Fascial System;* Luigi Stecco and John V. Basmajan, *Fasical Maninpulation for Musculoskeletal Pain.*

[148] LM Tham et al, "Cupping: From a Biomechanical Perspective," *Journal of Biomechanics,* 2006.

[149] Nowicki A, Dobruch-Sobczak K, "Introduction to ultrasound elastography," *Journal of Ultrasonography,* 2016;16(65):113-124.doi:10.15557/JoU.2016.0013.

[150] Michael J. Alter, *Science of Flexibility*, 82.

[151] Elham Ettari et al, "Proprioceptive Neuromuscular Facilitation," California State University—Sacramento, available online at http://www. csus.edu/indiv/m/mckeoughd/pt224/litreviewtopics/pnfpresentation.pps

[152] Lee Burton and Heidi Brigham, "Proprioceptive Neuromuscular Facilitation: The Foundation of Functional Training," July 7, 2013, available online at http://www. functionalmovement.com/articles/Screening/2013-07-04_proprioceptive_neuromuscular_facilitation_the_foundation_of_functional_training

[153] Kayla Hindle, "Proprioceptive Neuromuscular Facilitation (PNF): Its Mechanisms and Effects on Range of Motion and Muscular Function," *Journal of Human Kinetics*, March 2012.

[154] Greg Roskopf, "What is MAT?" *Muscle Activation. com,* available online at https://muscleactivation. com/about-us/what-is-mat/

[155] Jason Masek, "Femoroacetabular Impingement: Mechanisms, Diagnosis and Treatment Options Using Postural Restoration. Part 2," *SportEx,* June 2015.

[156] Claire Frank et al, "Dynamic Neuromuscular Stabilization and Sports Rehabilitation," *International Journal of Sports Physical Therapy,* February 2013.

[157] Pavel Kolar, "Dynamic Neuromuscular Stabilization (DNS) According to Kolar: A Developmental Kinesiology Approach," Rehabilitation Prague School, www.rehabps.com.

[158] Dr. Shirley Sahrmann, "Diagnosis and Treatment of Movement System Impairment Syndromes, parts B and C," Washington University in St. Louis School of Medicine.

[159] Shirley Sahrmann, "Diagnosis and Treatment of Movement System Impairment Syndromes, part B."

[160] Shirley Sahrmann, "Diagnosis and Treatment of Movement System Impairment Syndromes, part A."

[161] Mark Comerford and Sarah Mottram, *Kinetic Control: The Management of Uncontrolled Movement*, 3-5.

[162] Shirley Sahrmann, *Diagnosis and Treatment of Movement System Impairment Syndromes*, 219-221.

[163] Gray Cook, "It is All About Motor Control," www.graycook.com.

[164] Warrick McNeill, "Neurodynamics for Pilates Teachers," *Journal of Bodywork and Movement*, 2012.

[165] Allan Menezes, *The Complete Guide to Joseph H. Pilates' Techniques of Physical Conditioning*, 33.

[166] Sureeporn Phrompaet et al, "Effects of Pilates Training on Lumbo-Pelvic Stability and Flexibility," *Asian Journal of Sports Medicine*, March 2011.

[167] Karina M. Cancelliero-Gaiad et al, "Respiratory Pattern of Diaphragmatic Breathing and Pilates Breathing in COPD Subjects," *Brazilian Journal of Physical Therapy*, July 2014.

[168] Engel GL. "The need for a new medical model: a challenge for biomedicine," *Psychodynamic Psychiatry*, 2012;40(3):377–396

[169] Covassin T, Beidler E, Ostrowski J, Wallace J, "Psychosocial Aspects of Rehabilitation in Sports," *Clinics in Sports Medicine*, 2015;34(2):199-212.doi:10.1016/j.csm.2014.12.004.

[170] Clement D, Granquist MD, Arvinen-Barrow MM, "Psychosocial Aspects of Athletic Injuries as Perceived by Athletic Trainers," *Journal of Athletic Training*, 2013;48(4):512-521.doi:10.4085/1062-6050-48.3.21.

[171] Ibid.

[172] Hamson-Utley JJ, Martin S, Walters J, "Athletic trainers' and physical therapists' perceptions of the effectiveness of psychological skills within sport injury rehabilitation programs," *Journal of Athletic Training*, 2008;43(3):258.

[173] Podlog L, Dionigi R, "Coach strategies for addressing psychosocial challenges during the return to sport from injury," *Journal of Sports Sciences*, 2010;28(11):1197-1208.doi:10.1080/02640414.2010.487873.

[174] Arvinen-Barrow M, Massey WV, Hemmings B, "Role of Sport Medicine Professionals in Addressing Psychosocial Aspects of Sport-Injury Rehabilitation: Professional Athletes' Views," *Journal of Athletic Training*, 2014;49(6):764-772.

[175] Ibid.

[176] L. Judge et al, "Perceived Social Support from Strength and Conditioning Coaches among Injured Student Athletes," *Journal of Strength and Conditioning Research*, 2012.

[177] Laura Simon, Igor Elman and David Borsook, "Psychological Processing in Chronic Pain: A Neural Systems Approach," *Neuroscience Behavior Review*, December 2013.

[178] Ibid.

[179] Gordon Waddell, Mary Newton, Iain Henderson, Douglas Somerville and Chris J. Main, "A Fear-Avoidance Beliefs Questionnaire (FABQ) and the role of fear-avoidance beliefs in chronic low back pain and disability," *Pain*, 52 (1993) 157–168,166.

[180] D. Clement et al, "Psychosocial Aspects of Athletic Injuries as Perceived by Athletic Trainers," *Journal of Athletic Training*, 2013.

[181] Bond K, Ospina MB, Hooton N et al, "Defining a complex intervention: The development of demarcation criteria for 'meditation,'" *Psychology of Religion and Spirituality*, 2009;1(2):129-137.doi:10.1037/a0015736.

[182] Carter KS, Iii RC, "Breath-based meditation: A mechanism to restore the physiological and cognitive reserves for optimal human performance," *World Journal of Clinical Cases*, 2016;4(4):99.doi:10.12998/wjcc.v4.i4.99.

[183] Brown RP, Gerbarg PL, "Sudarshan Kriya yogic breathing in the treatment of stress, anxiety, and depression: part I-neurophysiologic model," *Journal of Alternative Complementary Medicine*, 2005;11(1):189–201.

[184] KS Carter, "Breath-Based Meditation: A Mechanism to Restore the Physiological and Cognitive Reserves for Optimal Human Performance," *World Journal of Clinical Cases*, 2016.

[185] RP Brown and PL Gerbarg, "Sudarshan Kriya Yogic Breathing in the Treatment of Stress, Anxiety, and Depression: Part I-Neurophysiologic Model," *Journal of Alternative Complementary Medicine*, 2005.

[186] Jim Afremow, *The Champion's Comeback,* 175.

[187] Sandler S, "The physiology of soft tissue massage," *Journal of Bodywork and Movement Therapies*, 1999;3(2):118–122.

[188] Smith LL, Keating MN, Holbert D et al, "The effects of athletic massage on delayed onset muscle soreness, creatine kinase, and neutrophil count: a preliminary report," *Journal of Orthopaedic and Sports Physical Therapy*, 1994;19(2):93–99.

[189] Ogai R, Yamane M, Matsumoto T, Kosaka M, "Effects of petrissage massage on fatigue and exercise performance following intensive cycle pedalling," *British Journal of Sports Medicine*, 2008;42(10):534-538.doi:10.1136/bjsm.2007 044396.

[190] Breger Stanton DE, Lazaro R, MacDermid JC, "A Systematic Review of the Effectiveness of Contrast Baths," *Journal of Hand Therapy*, 2009;22(1):57-70.doi:10.1016/j.jht.2008.08.001.

[191] Higgins T, Cameron M, Climstein M, "Evaluation of passive recovery, cold water immersion, and contrast baths for recovery, as measured by game performances markers, between two simulated games of rugby union," *Journal of Strength and Conditioning Research*, June 2012:1.doi:10.1519/JSC.0b013e31825c32b9.

[192] Duffield R, Edge J, Merrells R et al, "The effects of compression garments on intermittent exercise performance and recovery on consecutive days," *International Journal of Sports Physiology and Performance*, 2008;3(4):454-468.

[193] Duffield R, Cannon J, King M, "The effects of compression garments on recovery of muscle performance following high-intensity sprint and plyometric exercise," *Journal of Science and Medicine in Sport*, 2010;13(1):136-140.doi:10.1016/j.jsams.2008.10.006.

[194] Duffield R, Portus M, "Comparison of three types of full-body compression garments on throwing and repeat-sprint performance in cricket players," *British Journal of Sports Medicine*, 2007;41(7):409-414; discussion414.doi:10.1136/bjsm.2006.033753.

[195] Lombardi G, Ziemann E, Banfi G, "Whole-Body Cryotherapy in Athletes: From Therapy to Stimulation. An Updated Review of the Literature," *Frontiers in Physiology*, 2017;8.doi:10.3389/fphys.2017.00258.

[196] Dr. Patrick Dougherty, "Somatosensory Systems," available online at http://neuroscience.uth.tmc.edu/s2/chapter02.html

[197] Riemann BL, Lephart SM, "The sensorimotor system, part I: the physiologic basis of functional joint stability," *Journal of Athletic Training*, 2002;37(1):71.

[198] "Facts About Perception," *National Geographic,* September 2011.

[199] "The Human Balance System," Vestibular Disorders Association, available online at http://vestibular.org/understanding-vestibular-disorder/human-balance-system

[200] Lenore Herget, "Concussion: Visuo-Vestibular Rehab," Massachusetts General Hospital, available online at https://www.childrenshospital.org/~/media/landing-pages/alt-tests/concussion-conference/new-concussion-pdfs/hergetconcussionvisuovestibular-rehab.ashx?la=en

[201] Ibid.

[202] Michael Higgins, *Therapeutic Exercise: From Theory to Practice,* 274.

[203] Gill Connell and Cheryl McCarthy, *A Moving Child Is a Learning Child: How the Body Teaches the Brain to Think*, 48.

[204] Pamela Jeter et al, "Ashtanga-Based Yoga Therapy Increases the Sensory Contribution to Postural Stability in Visually-Impaired Persons at Risk for Falls as Measured by the Wii Balance Board," *PLOS One,* June 2015.

[205] Catherine Kerr et al, "Mindfulness Starts with the Body: Somatosensory Attention and Top-Down Modulation of Cortical Alpha Rhythms in Mindfulness Meditation," *Frontiers in Human Neuroscience,* February 2013.

[206] Bernie Clark, "An Introduction to Yin Yoga," www.yinyoga.com.

[207] Shrier I, "Does stretching improve performance?: a systematic and critical review of the literature," *Clinical Journal of Sports Medicine*, 2004;14(5):267.

[208] Ibid.

[209] Ikuo Homma and Yuri Masaoka, "Breathing Rhythms and Emotions," *Experimental Physiology,* September 2008.

[210] Rachel Vickery, "The Effect of Breathing Pattern Retraining on Performance in Competitive Cyclists," Auckland University of Technology thesis, 2007.

[211] Scott Lucett, "Dysfunctional Breathing and Its Effects on the Kinetic Chain," *National Academy of Sports Medicine,* March 2013.

[212] Pavel Kolar et al, "Postural Function of the Diaphragm in Persons With and Without Chronic Low Back Pain," *Journal of Orthopedic and Sports Physical Therapy,* April 2012.

[213] Tania Clifton-Smith and Janet Rowley, "Breathing Pattern Disorders and Physiotherapy: Inspiration for Our Profession," *Physical Therapy Reviews*, 2011.

[214] Brown R, Gerbarg P, "Sudarshan Kriya Yogic Breathing in the Treatment of Stress, Anxiety, and Depression: Part I—Neurophysiologic Model," *The Journal of Alternative and Complementary Medicine*, 2005;11(1):189-201.doi:10.1089/acm.2005.11.189.

[215] Carter KIII R, "Breath-based meditation: A mechanism to restore the physiological and cognitive reserves for optimal human performance," *World Journal of Clinical Cases*, 2016;4(4):99.doi:10.12998/wjcc.v4.i4.99.

[216] Sarah Jamieson, "Dysfunctional Breathing Patterns: Breath Changes Movement," *Vancouver YogaReview.com*, February 2014.

[217] Obayashi H, Urabe Y, Yamanaka Y, Okuma R, "Effects of respiratory-muscle exercise on spinal curvature," *Journal of Sport Rehabilitation*, 2012;21(1):63–68.

[218] Alison McConnel, "Anatomy and Physiology of Muscles Involved in Breathing," *Human Kinetics*, available online at http://www.humankinetics. com/excerpts/excerpts/ learn-the-anatomy-and-physiology-of-the-muscles-involved-in-breathing.

[219] Jason Masek, "Breathing's Influence On Upper Quarter Dysfunction," NATA Annual Meeting and Clinical Symposia, June 27, 2013.

[220] Nicole Nelson, "Diaphragmatic Breathing: The Foundation of Core Stability, *Strength and Conditioning Journal*, 2012.

[221] Sir Charles Sherrington, *The Integrative Action of the Nervous System*, 1906.

[222] Clare Frank, "Dynamic Neuromuscular Stabilization and Sports Rehabilitation," *International Journal of Sports Physical Therapy*, February 2013.

[223] Karl Lewit, "Lessons for the Future," Internal Musculoskeletal Medicine, 30(3), 2008, 133-140.

[224] Karl Lewit, "Chain Reactions in the Locomotor System," *The Journal of Orthopedic Medicine*, 21(1), 1999, 52-57.

[225] Ferrante MA, Ferrante ND, "The Thoracic Outlet Syndromes: Part 1. Overview of the Thoracic Outlet Syndromes and Review of True Neurogenic Outlet Syndrome," *Muscle Nerve*, 2017, 55:782-793.

[226] SJ Mulholland et al, "Activities of Daily Living in Non-Western Cultures: Range of Motion Requirements for Hip and Knee Joint Implants, "*International Journal of Rehabilitation Research*, 2001.

[227] A Hemmerich et al, "Hip, Knee, and Ankle Kinematics of High Range of Motion Activities of Daily Living," *Journal of Orthopedic Research*, April 2006.

[228] Saeed Rad, "Impact of Ethnic Habits on Defecographic Measurements," *Archive of Iranian Medicine*, 2002.

[229] Page P, Frank C, Lardner R, *Assessment And Treatment Of Muscle Imbalance, 1st edition*, Champaign, IL, Human Kinetics, 2010.

[230] Phil Hoffman, "Conclusions Drawn From a Comparative Study of the Feet of Barefooted and Shoe-Wearing Peoples, *American Journal of Orthopedic Surgery*, 1905, 105-136.

[231] SK Lynn, "Differences in Static and Dynamic Balance Task Performance after Four Weeks of Intrinsic Foot Muscle Training," *Journal of Sports Rehabilitation*, November 2012.

[232] Doug Richie, "How To Treat Hallux Rigidus in Runners," *Podiatry Today*, March 2009.

[233] Paul Scherer, "Understanding The Biomechanical Effects of Hallux Limitus," *Podiatry Today*, August 2007.

[234] Beach P, *Muscles And Meridians, 1st ed*, Edinburgh, Churchill Livingstone, 2010.

[235] Craig Payne, "The Windlass Mechanism of the Foot," *Running Research Junkie*, April 2013, available online at http://www.runresearchjunkie.com/the-windlass-mechanism-foot/.

[236] Michael Sullivan et al, "Catastrophizing and Pain Perception in Sports Participants," *Journal of Applied Sport Psychology, 2000.*

[237] Kendall F, *Muscles: Testing and Function, with Posture and Pain, 5th edition*, Wolters Kluwer, 2005.

[238] Francis G. O'Connor, *ACSM's Sports Medicine: A Comprehensive Review*, 741.

[239] JM Wilson et al, "The Effects of Endurance, Strength, and Power Training on Muscle Fiber Type Shifting." *Journal of Strength and Conditioning Research*, June 2012.

[240] An Bogaerts, "Power Plate Training Increases Strength and Muscle Mass in Older Men," *Journal of Gerontology*, 2007.

[241] Jordan MJ, Norris SR, Smith DJ, Herzog W, others, "Vibration training: an overview of the area, training consequences, and future considerations," *Journal of Strength and Conditioning Research*, 2005;19(2):459–466.

[242] Nicholas A. Burd et al, "Muscle time under tension during resistance exercise stimulates differential muscle protein sub-fractional synthetic responses in men," *Journal of Physiology*, 2010.

[243] QT Tran et al, "The Effects of Varying Time Under Tension and Volume Load on Acute Neuromuscular Response," *European Journal of Applied Physiology*, November 2006.

[244] VS Husby et al, "Early Postoperative Maximal Strength Training Improves Work Efficiency 6-12 Months after Osteoarthritis-Induced Total Hip Arthroplasty in Patients Younger Than 60 Years," *American Journal of Physical Medicine and Rehabilitation*, April 2010.

[245] LJ Distefano, "Comparison of Integrated and Isolated Training on Performance Measures and Neuromuscular Control," *Journal of Strength and Conditioning Research,* April 2013.

[246] Josh McHugh, "Get Your Body Back to Age 20," *Men's Journal.*

[247] Benjamin Rosenblatt, "Planning a Performance Programme," *High Performance Training for Sports,* Dan Lewindon and David Joyce, editors, 248-249.

[248] DL Hoover, "Periodization and Physical Therapy: Bridging the Gap Between Training and Rehabilitation," *Physical Therapy in Sport,* March 2016.

[249] Glenn Stewart, "Minimizing the Interference Effect," *High Performance Training for Sports,* Dan Lewindon and David Joyce, editors, 246-247.

[250] J Mikkola et al, "Neuromuscular and Cardiovascular Adaptations During Concurrent Strength and Endurance Training in Untrained Men," *International Journal of Sports Medicine,* September 2012.

[251] JM Wilson et al, "Concurrent Training: a Meta-Analysis Examining Interference of Aerobic and Resistance Exercises," *Journal of Strength and Conditioning Research,* August 2012.

[252] Nick Winkelman, "The TEC Model: Deceleration," *EXOS,* available online at http://education.athletesperformance.com/articles-2/EXOS-tec-model/the-tec-model-deceleration/.

[253] Cory Toth, "Injuries to the Nervous System Occurring in Sport and Recreation: A Systematic Review," *Critical Reviews in Physical and Rehabilitation Medicine,* 2012.

[254] MA Britto, "Analysis of Jumping-Landing Manoeuvers after Different Speed Performances in Soccer Players," *Journal of Kinanthropometry and Human Performance,* November 2015.

[255] Abdolhamid Daneshjoo et al, "Analysis of Jumping-Landing Manoeuvers after Different Speed Performances in Soccer Players," *PLOS One,* November 2015.

[256] Timothy Hewett, "Why Women Have an Increased Risk of an ACL Injury," AAOS.

[257] Thomas Baechle and Roger Earle, *Essentials of Strength Training and Conditioning, 3rd edition,* 414.

[258] Nicole Chimera et al, "Effects of Plyometric Training on Muscle-Activation Strategies and Performance in Female Athletes," *Journal of Athletic Training,* January 2004.

[259] Bill Horan, *High Performance Sports Conditioning,* 152-153.

[260] Y Kawakami et al, "In Vivo Muscle Fibre Behaviour During Counter-Movement Exercise in Humans Reveals a Significant Role for Tendon Elasticity," *Journal of Physiology,* 2002.

[261] Bruce Reider et al, *Orthopaedic Rehabilitation of the Athlete: Getting Back in the Game,* 57.

[262] Kawakami, Y., Muraoka, T., Ito, S., Kanehisa, H. and Fukunaga, T. (2002), In vivo muscle fibre behaviour during counter-movement exercise in humans reveals a significant role for tendon elasticity, *The Journal of Physiology,* 540: 635–646.

[263] Giulio Sergio Roi, "Return to Competition Following Athletic Injury: Sports Rehabilitation as a Whole," *Medicina de l'Esport,* 2010.

[264] Mario Bizzini et al, "Suggestions From the Field for Return to Sports Participation Following Anterior Cruciate Ligament Reconstruction: Soccer," *Journal of Orthopedic and Sports Physical Therapy,* April 2012.

[265] Raphael Brandon, "Rehabilitation Process—So What Exactly is the Coach Meant to Do During The Rehabilitation Period? Here are a Few Pointers," http://www.sportsinjurybulletin.com/.

[266] Damien Farrow et al, "Skill and Physiological Demands of Open and Closed Training Drills in Australian Football," *International journal of Sports Science and Coaching,* December 2008.

[267] Tyler Kepner, "Perry Hill Delivers a Simple Message for a Complex Task," *New York Times,* February 26, 2016.

[268] Joseph B. Myers et al, "The Role of the Sensorimotor System in the Athletic Shoulder," *Journal of Athletic Training,* 2000.

[269] BJ Kissel, "Breaking Down the Art of the QB Audible," *Bleacher Report,* July 2013, available online at http://bleacherreport.com/articles/1716979-breaking-down-the-art-of-the-qb-audible.

[270] "Training Modes for Speed," *World Rugby,* available online at http://www.irbsandc.com/.

[271] Michael Lawrence et al, "The Effect of Load on Movement Coordination During Sled Towing," American Society of Biomechanics National Conference, 2012.

[272] Bruce Reider et al, *Orthopaedic Rehabilitation of the Athlete: Getting Back in the Game,* 347-348.

[273] James Rheuben Andrews et al, *Physical Rehabilitation of the Injured Athlete,* 62-63.

[274] Tatiana Dobrescu, "The Role of Non-verbal Communication in the Coach-Athlete Relationship," *Procedia–Social and Behavioral Sciences,* September 2014.

[275] Allison Belger, "Coping with Injury: The Psychology of Being Sidelined," *CrossFit Invictus,* available online at https://www.crossfitinvictus.com/blog/coping-with-injury-the-psychology-of-being-sidelined/.

[276] Ty Shalter, "Are NFL Athletes Playing a Dangerous Game with Too-Fast ACL Returns?" *Bleacher Report,* February 2015.

[277] William Kraemer et al, "Recovery From Injury in Sport: Considerations in the Transition From Medical Care to Performance Care," *Sports Health,* 2009.

# INDEX

# ABOUT THE AUTHOR

Sue is the Founder of Structure & Function Education and Falsone Consulting, along with being an Associate Professor in the Athletic Training Programs at A.T. Still University.

Growing up in Buffalo, New York, Sue stayed local to attend Daemen College, where she obtained her bachelor's degree in physical therapy. From there she moved to North Carolina to begin working in outpatient orthopedics, where she went back to school at the University of North Carolina Chapel Hill to pursue a master's degree in Human Movement Science with a Concentration in Sports Medicine.

After graduate school, Sue moved to Arizona, where she began working at Athletes' Performance, developing the physical therapy program within the performance program. It is at Athletes' Performance where she began her focus on Bridging the Gap from Rehab to Performance, working closely with the performance and nutritional teams to create an integrative experience for all athletes. She spent 13 years there, creating, developing, and cultivating this craft.

During her time at Athletes' Performance she began working for the LA Dodgers, first as a consultant and the moving into the Head Athletic Trainer position for the Major League club. After six years, she left the Dodgers and eventually became the Head of Athletic Training and Sport Performance for the US Men's National Soccer team.

After she left US Soccer, she began her own education and consulting business, as well as joining the staff at A.T Still University.

For over two decades, Sue has immersed herself in the culture, education, and advancement of the athletic training, physical therapy, and strength and conditioning professions. She aims to provide the highest quality education for all types of health care professionals.

Sue resides in Phoenix, AZ, with her beloved black and tan dachshund, Richard.

Made in the USA
Coppell, TX
19 December 2020